Nitya Living Cookbook

Seasonal, Local, Vegetarian Recipes

by Lydia Nitya Griffith

Copyright © 2021
Lydia "Nitya" Griffith
All Rights Reserved

ISBN 978-0-9905505-3-2

This is an updated, expanded edition of
Nitya's previous cookbook titled *Yoga with Nitya Cookbook*,
ISBN 978-0-9905505-2-5, Copyright © 2016.

Learn more about Nitya Living online at
www.NityaLiving.com

Acknowledgments

Front Cover Photo: Lula Fueglein, one of Nitya's students since the age of five, is an enthusiastic consumer and preparer of Nitya's Yoga Camp cuisine.

Page ix: Lilly Lynch (pictured) enjoyed preparing recipes from Nitya's first cookbook edition.

Page 81: The Yogi Yum-Yums snack photo courtesy of Miranda "Prasana" Yanez, Nitya's student since age 4, who is now in college.

Back Cover Photo: Candace Benn with her daughter Jayda preparing a meal for the camp kids. Candace is one of several certified Nitya Living Kids Yoga teachers.

Editor, Designer: Ian F. Wesley

Special Thanks to all the Nitya Living Camp kids and Yoga students. Thank you for inspiring us all to live more consciously and healthfully.

Introduction

Why Did I Write This Book?

I want to inspire you to make a notable shift in the way your family eats and the relationship you have with food. It is the most important thing you do every day—nourish your body so that you can have the strength and vitality to get through your day. Over many years of feeding campers at the Nitya Living Summer Camp, the kids have begged me to write this cookbook so their moms and dads will know how to cook the fabulous meals and snacks we provide. We have turned many picky eaters into adventurous eaters.

I have been teaching yoga to kids and teens since 2005 throughout the Richmond community as well as hosting workshops along the East Coast. One thing I have noticed when I teach in schools and daycares is that the foods provided are not conducive to focus and vitality. What a travesty! The behavior of the children could be drastically improved if the foods they were served were alive, nourishing, and far less processed. So much of what I have directly witnessed students consuming is highly processed and full of white flour, sugar, grease, salt and colorings. Sure, it tastes good, but it is hardly nourishing or healthful, despite being approved by the FDA, state regulators, and local school boards. We have a *long* way to go before we see progressive change in that area when we have a government that recognizes tomato paste on pizza as a vegetable serving and rebukes the idea of labeling genetically modified organisms (GMOs).

Studies have demonstrated that when the food offered in schools changes to more fresh fruits and vegetables, and less processed junk, attention goes up, the rate of violence goes down, sickness and absences are fewer, and overall performance increases. The 2017 Nutrition Policy Institute study found that better quality school lunches averaged a 4 percent boost in academic achievement. That's half a letter grade for the whole student body!

My dream is to see every school growing some of their own food with an organic garden that is integrated into the science curriculum, so children have hands-on experience gardening from seed, to plant, to food on the table. My other dream is to see every family having dinner together 3–4 nights a week at minimum—to see everyone giving thanks in a mindful

INTRODUCTION

blessing, sharing the same meal, conversing about their day, and *being a family* (with no distractions from cell phones, television, or other devices). Every family should attempt to grow a garden, too—even a windowsill herb garden or a raised garden in pots on the patio. How you feed your family and yourself should be one of your top priorities, not something to shove to the side as a great inconvenience. Fast, processed meals might be convenient, but are no substitute for meals made with fresh, vital, living ingredients and the satisfaction brought by preparing them yourself.

My Food Journey

As a young teen in high school I became very interested in nutrition, and that was my original career goal until I found out I'd have to go to medical school (which was not an option for me). Later, in my early twenties, I began reading about the devastation of the rainforests and how beef was one of the main causes of deforestation. So, I gave up eating beef and became a pretty radical environmentalist, joining in protests and working for Clean Water Action. Then, in my early thirties, I started a relationship with a Buddhist who was vegetarian. The main reason for eliminating meat from my diet then became spiritual. I would say that over the decades I always aimed to eat a healthy diet—never a fan of microwaving frozen dinners, eating fast food or bingeing on junk food.

In 2006, I read a book that changed my life and the way I ate forever: *An Omnivore's Dilemma* by Michael Pollan. This book intelligently argues *both sides* of the "eat meat/don't eat meat" debate. The reading of this book coincided with my becoming an Integral Yoga teacher, which also promotes a vegetarian diet as part of the practice of *saucha* (cleanliness-purity) and *ahimsa* (non-violence). In essence, by eating a clean, pure diet, you are better able to do the Hatha yoga poses, sit in meditation, and lead a calmer, more peaceful life. I then went on to read Barbara Kingsolver's *Animal, Vegetable, Miracle,* which is a nonfiction book about her own family's quest to spend one year eating seasonally and locally.

After that wonderfully inspiring read, I thought to myself, "Why can't *I* do this?" And then I wondered, "Why can't I make this *my* lifestyle?" So, ever since then, I have enjoyed living a very different way from most people, but I am determined to inspire as many people as I can to try to eat a diet that is vegetarian, sustainable, GMO/chemical-free, locally sourced, and

INTRODUCTION

seasonal. It is surprisingly doable and it does not require any more effort on your part, just some planning.

As motivated as I already was from my reading, I then watched several mind-blowing documentaries that really brought all I knew into a very graphic image I could not ignore. The excuse of "this is just how I've always eaten and I'm not going to change" didn't cut it anymore. I couldn't excuse causing unnecessary and horrific suffering to countless animals and harm to the environment, not to mention the consequences to my family's health. As a global community, it's time for us all, starting with myself, to grow up and be responsible, compassionate stewards of all of life on earth, including the earth herself. The documentaries I saw were *Food Inc., Forks over Knives, The Beautiful Truth*, and *Thrive*. A couple great ones for kids are *OMG GMO, That Sugar Film,* and *What's on My Plate?* Great books for kids are *That's Why We Don't Eat Animals* and *Vegan is Love*, both by Ruby Roth. Plus, she has a kids' cookbook called *Help Yourself Cookbook for Kids*.

What I know is this—our food consumption habits and traditions are poisoning us and play a major role in skyrocketing rates of obesity, diabetes, heart disease, cancer, and even neurological disorders, including the pandemic of ADD/ADHD. These conditions are largely preventable or reversible with a clean, pure diet. Dr. Dean Ornish famously proved this in his bestselling book *Reversing Heart Disease*. He was a friend and disciple of my guru, Swami Satchidananda, and spoke many times at Satchidananda Ashram Yogaville.

I recommend Sri Swami Satchidananda's book, *The Healthy Vegetarian*, and anything written by Dean Ornish, Michael Pollan, or Jamie Oliver.

Seasonal Changes. Due to climate change, the seasons are changing. Some years, summer bleeds into October and even into early November when there are still green tomatoes, peppers, and squash growing. It would seem winter and fall are shortening, expanding our warmer seasons and changing how nature responds. Eating according to the seasons brings you into harmony with your environment. As the weather fluctuates, affecting what is growing when, we also need to be mindful of what might be available at the farmers' market from week to week.

INTRODUCTION

Is This Doable and How?

Know when and where fresh, seasonal foods are available. If you don't have a plan, you might have a rough start. I first embarked on eating seasonal/local foods during a winter season, and by the time spring arrived I never wanted to eat another sweet potato again in my life! When asparagus arrived in late April, I gorged on those long spindly green delights voraciously. Next came the spring greens and the return of salad days. By May strawberries were available, though like asparagus only for about two months. That summer I began what is now a ritual, putting up the bounty of summer's harvest. It's a matter of reserving a weekend in July or early August to can and freeze (see the "Putting Up for Winter" section). As messy as the process is, it is a labor of love from which you reap rewards all winter long.

The options for what you can do with all that's available in summertime are endless. As the peaches, corn, and berries finish their season mid-August, a wave of root vegetables arrives—beets, potatoes, carrots, and eggplant. Depending on the weather we might have tomatoes, squash, and zucchini into October and even early November.

How do you know what's in season? Sure, I listed them in the Table of Contents (categorized by season), but *it's essential that you become a regular farmers' market shopper.* Here in the Richmond area we have so many farmers' markets and farmstands offering abundances of fruits, veggies, eggs, honey, yogurt, cheese, bread, and herbs year-round. The dead of winter is really my only challenge but freezing and canning keeps meals diverse enough to be interesting.

Know what you're eating. I buy very little from traditional grocery stores. Most of what you find in a supermarket is not necessarily food and doesn't belong in a healthy diet, despite the fact that it's been *engineered* to taste good.

I am often amazed by the number of people I know who do not realize what GMOs are or the great and real risks GMO poses to the future of food and our health. Here's how the Non-GMO Project defines them:

> "GMOs (genetically modified organisms) are organisms whose genetic material has been artificially manipulated in a laboratory through genetic engineering, or GE. This relatively new science creates unstable combinations of plant, animal, bacterial and viral

INTRODUCTION

genes that do not occur in nature or through traditional crossbreeding methods."

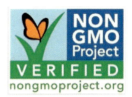

Check out their website (nongmoproject.org) to learn about what ingredients contain GMO and more fascinating information. Look for foods that bear the NGP Verified seal (right). Bottom line: *avoid GMO foods* (which often translates to: "avoid highly processed foods"). Lead paint may taste good, but we know not to eat it. Just because something tastes good doesn't mean you or your family should eat it.

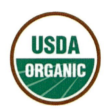

While shopping for groceries, also look for the labels that assure you that a product is Certified Organic. If it's not organic, you're eating "acceptable levels" of pesticides, petroleum, and hormones (in addition to the toxins you're already exposed to in non-food products, buildings, clothes, and your environment).

I am gluten-sensitive (as are a great many people with digestive, joint, and inflammatory issues), so we look for "GF" symbols when it comes to pastas, breads, and even sauces. Gluten is a protein found in wheat, barley and rye, but food manufacturers extract and use gluten as a thickening agent, binder, and stabilizer in a tremendous array of processed foods.

Additional motivations for eating locally grown foods are the benefit to your local economy and the reduction of pollution. Non-local foods require extra petroleum, preservatives, processing and packaging for transport over long distances. That's a lot of waste to create for foods that are less fresh and vital. Similarly, eating seasonally is not only natural, but requires less processing and transport than "unseasonal" foods. The more we eat locally and seasonally, the more we sustain our local economy and the less we support the centralization of the food industry into mega corporations which employ the worst practices.

Know what you're drinking. The number one drink you should hydrate yourself with throughout your day is *water*, and little else. Remember, we are water beings living on a water planet. Your body needs water to function properly. Children do not *need* milk (that's an old paradigm from the 1950s). What other mammals regularly consume milk past infancy,

INTRODUCTION

much less from other species? *None!* It's unnatural and leads to infections, bone problems, and auto-immune disorders, including allergies. The average American child drinks 104 quarts of cow's milk every year. In fact, scientific studies show that drinking milk actually strips calcium from bones. In regions of the world where little to no milk or dairy is consumed, Japan for example, there is hardly any osteoporosis or breast cancer. Check out Save Our Bones online for more on this and watch *Forks over Knives*. While I do include some butter and cheese in this cookbook (which are better tolerated by most than milk itself), non-dairy options are provided in most cases. Dairy consumption is entirely unnecessary and should be done sparingly and with care that it was produced humanely, organically, and responsibly.

Know what you're supporting. You've heard it said, "You vote with your dollar." This is *so* very true, and I am mindful about what I buy and who/what I am supporting with my shopping habits. Being a consumer who supports local farmers, local businesses, and ethical, sustainable practices is to be an advocate for the environment, my families' health, and the future of food for generations to come.

Seriously, at what point in recent history did it become "reasonable" for people to have no clue what's in their food, where it comes from, or how it impacts the world our children will inherit? If you think about it, seasonal-local-organic isn't a radical diet whatsoever. It's how all human beings ate until less than a century ago. Rather, it is our society that has become radical in its industrialized food-producing and mass consumption practices. It is past time to turn back toward sane living.

We have a moral obligation to eat this way.

How to Begin

At the end of each week I sit down and write the coming week's menu. This exercise takes no more than a few minutes and is nice to do with your partner and even the kids. Consider what you do have in the fridge and cupboards, what meals you'd like to eat, and everyone's schedule. With that information build the menu, and from the menu your grocery list. This way your shopping is more efficient, and less food is wasted. I tend to cook dinners with leftovers in mind, which makes lunches that much simpler, too.

Introduction

Organizing your life in this way brings so much more ease around mealtime. When you know on a busy day that you are having spaghetti with a salad for dinner, you have one less thing to think about. On a less busy day you have time to make something more involved, like vegetable lasagna. You also save a lot of money by not buying things you don't need and eating out less often.

Thank you for caring enough about your family's well-being to give seasonal, local, vegetarian, GMO/chemical-free eating a try. You will be amazed at how incredibly clean your body will feel and how your health will improve, with a stronger immune system, easier digestion and elimination, and a calmer disposition. It doesn't take any more of your time, and if anything, it should prove to be easier. You just have to get organized and make it part of your routine and ultimately how you live.

I've organized this book so you have *complete meals* with each recipe. I trust that you know better than to feed your family and the planet chemicals, so I did not denote organic for *every* ingredient. No excuses that it costs too much, because when you really look at the equation, you are spending a lot less on future medical expenses while spending a bit more on really, really good food.

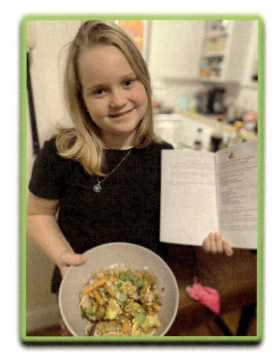

INDEX OF RECIPES

Index of Recipes
(Table of Contents)

The recipes in this book are divided according to the four seasons, with additional sections for "Meals for Any Season," and "Breakfast and Snacks," plus a section on "Putting Up for Winter" (yes, like squirrels). You can plan your weekly menu from the current season and supplement it with the Meals for Any Season.

Most of these recipes will easily feed a family of four, usually with enough remaining for leftovers.

Camp favorites are marked with a heart (♥).

WINTER
(DECEMBER THROUGH MARCH)

What's in Season: *Root veggies, potatoes, sweet potatoes, Brussels sprouts, beets, carrots, chard, kale, collards, and spinach.*

Suggestion: I make a large pot of soup every weekend in winter to enjoy for lunches or quick leftovers during the week.

African Peanut Soup with Gluten-Free Corn Bread	2
Cream of Cashew Soup with Roasted Sweet Potato Chips	3
Minestrone Soup	4
French Lentil Soup with Roasted Potatoes	6
Black Bean Soup with Cheesy Quesadillas	7
Kale-Garlic-Shiitake Soup with Carrot-Beet Ginger Salad	8
Layered No-Noodle Veggie Lasagna	10
Spaghetti Squash & Cheese with a Side of Steamed Greens	11
Roasted Root Medley with Goat Cheese & Pine Nuts	12
Creamy Carrot Ginger Soup	13
Thai Peanut Noodles with Steamed Chard	14

Index of Recipes

Scalloped Potatoes with Steamed Greens 15
Winter Root Soup 16

SPRING
(APRIL THROUGH JUNE)

What's in Season: Root veggies are waning while salad greens return with asparagus and strawberries.

Asparagus with Garlic Pasta 18
Indian Chickpea Curry on Rice 19
Spring Greens Salad with Quinoa 20
❤ Miss Nitya's Yoga Camp Salad Dressing 21
Sweet Potato and Black Bean Chili 22
Strawberry-Quinoa Salad 23
Chana Masala Stuffed Sweet Potatoes 24
Asparagus Soup 26
Chesapeake Bay Potato-Leek Soup 27

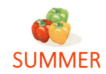

SUMMER
(JULY THROUGH SEPTEMBER)

What's in Season: Blueberries and blackberries arrive in July along with tomatoes, zucchini, yellow squash, okra, cucumbers, peppers, melons, peaches, and more salad greens.

Crabby Cakes with Sliced Heirloom Tomatoes and Potato Salad 30
Fried Okra on Pasta with Tomato Sauce 32
Loaded Salad with Lentils 33
Noodles with Summer Veggies in a Thai Peanut Sauce 34
Stuffed Red Peppers with Side Salad 36

INDEX OF RECIPES

Zu-Canoes 37

Gumbo with Sweet Cucumber Salad 38

Southwest Quinoa Salad 39

♥ Sesame Noodles with Squash and a Tomato Basil Salad 40

♥ Summer Veggie Soup with side of Roasted Potatoes 41

♥ Thai Noodles with Peanut Sauce 42

AUTUMN
(SEPTEMBER THROUGH NOVEMBER)

What's in Season: *Apples, pumpkin, squash, spinach, kale, chard, potatoes, carrots, beets, tomatoes, zucchini, onion, and eggplant.*

Italian Fried Eggplant 45

Shepherd's Pie 46

Raw Vegan Cheddar Cheese 47

Asian Rice Noodle Stir Fry 48

Fall Veggie Casserole 49

Fried Green Tomatoes Topped with Cheese on Pasta 50

Roasted Pumpkin on Rice 52

Roasted Brussels Sprouts 53

MEALS FOR ANY SEASON

♥ Rice & Black Beans with Salsa 56

Indian Kitchari with Cucumber Salad 57

♥ Aloo Tikki (Indian Potato Cakes) and Green Chutney 58

Tomato-Garlic Pasta 59

♥ Chicky Cakes with Roasted Potatoes 60

INDEX OF RECIPES

Portabella Mushroom Melt 61

Asian Stir Fry 62

♥ Chickpea Tacos 63

♥ Cheesy Quesadillas with Corn and Refried Black Beans 64

♥ Nachos 65

Barbecue Tofu or Tempeh with Roasted Veggies on Rice 66

Stuffed Baked Potatoes 67

Fried Rice 68

♥ Cold Veggie Pasta Salad 69

♥ Veggie Sushi 70

♥ Grandma Mary's Veggie Burgers 72

♥ Miso Soup with Fried Rice 73

Vegetarian Chili with Corn Bread 74

BREAKFAST & SNACKS

Breakfast at Ms. Nitya's (Homemade Granola and Hot Oatmeal).... 76

♥ Fruit Smoothie (dessert) 78

Green Juice Cleanse 79

Fruit Juice Cleanse 80

♥ Yogi Yum-Yums (snack) 81

Chickpea Poppers (snack) 82

♥ Ultimate Rice Cake (snack) 82

Fruit and Veggie Snacks 83

♥ Zucchini Muffins (dessert) 84

Sweet Potato Chips 85

♥ Strawberry Crumble (dessert) 86

xiii

INDEX OF RECIPES

PUTTING UP FOR WINTER

Freezing Ingredients	88
A Word About Canning	93

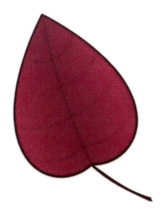

Recipes for Winter

RECIPES FOR WINTER

African Peanut Soup with Gluten-Free Corn Bread

2 cups chopped onion
1 Tbsp peanut oil
1 tsp fresh grated ginger root
1 cup chopped carrots
2 cups chopped sweet potato
4 cups vegetable stock or water
2 cups tomato juice
1 cup fresh ground peanut butter
1 cup chopped scallions or red onion

DIRECTIONS

Sauté onions in the oil until translucent.

Stir in the fresh ginger, add the carrots, sweet potatoes, and pour in the water or veggie stock (I use water).

Bring to a boil and simmer for 15 minutes or until the veggies are tender.

In a blender or food processor puree the vegetables with the cooking broth and the tomato juice.

Pour puree back in pot and stir in the peanut butter until smooth.

Serve topped with chopped scallions or red onion.

Variation: To ensure that there are leftovers to be enjoyed for lunches or quick dinners, I put in double the onions, carrots, sweet potatoes, and a large jar of my canned tomatoes. I also use about 1–2 *tablespoons* of grated ginger because I love it!

Corn Bread: Find a gluten-free, GMO-free, organic mix (like Red Mill, King Arthur, or Glutino brands). Prepare according to directions.

Kale Salad: Mix locally sourced kale with 1 tsp raw pressed ginger meat and shredded beet and carrot, then top with Miss Nitya's Dressing (page 21) for another wonderful side.

RECIPES FOR WINTER

Cream of Cashew Soup with Roasted Sweet Potato Chips

CREATED BY IAN FIRESTONE

**2 onions, medium, diced
½ stick butter or refined coconut oil
4 Tbsp olive oil
2 cups roasted cashews
2–3 Tbsp fresh ground peanut butter
2–3 Tbsp fresh ground almond butter
4 Tbsp nutritional yeast
6 cups water
1 tsp ground black pepper**

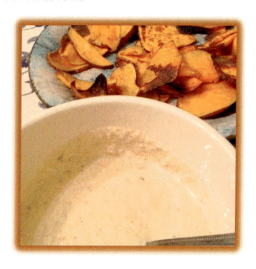

DIRECTIONS

Sauté black pepper and onions on medium heat in the butter and oil until onions are translucent. Add water and cashews and bring to a boil for 10 minutes to soften.

Remove from heat, add yeast and nut butters, then blend with a hand mixer (or a blender) until smooth.

On low heat simmer covered for 30 minutes. Uncover and stir frequently, scraping bottom with wooden spoon or silicone spatula for 10 minutes. Salt to taste.

Sweet Potato Chips

Slice 2 sweet potatoes thin, place on a cookie sheet, and toss in sea salt and vegetable oil.

Roast about 20 minutes in a 375° F oven. (Play with the temperature and time to get them just right—crispy and not-too-dark.)

RECIPES FOR WINTER

Minestrone Soup

2 large cloves crushed garlic
2 Tbsp olive oil
1 onion, large, chopped
1 16–24 oz jar canned tomatoes*
4 cups various chopped vegetables
   (whatever is in season—potatoes, carrots, peppers, green beans, okra, zucchini, or squash)
1–2 cups chopped carrot greens (optional)
6 cups water
1–2 cans black beans
   (or 1 cup dry beans, soaked overnight in 2 cups water)
2 cups gluten-free elbow macaroni
1–2 tsp balsamic vinegar (to taste)
Herbs: fresh rosemary, thyme, oregano, and/or basil to taste
salt and pepper to taste

*Use canned tomatoes from previous summer (see canning tips in back section); or, if summer, use 3–4 large tomatoes, pureed or diced.

DIRECTIONS

In a large pot add oil, garlic, and chopped onion on medium heat. Sauté until onion is translucent and slightly browned.

Add chopped vegetables and continue to sauté on medium heat for 8–12 minutes.

Deglaze the pan with a splash of balsamic vinegar (about 1 Tbsp) and using wooden spoon scrape bottom of pan to create a broth base.

Pour in water and canned (or fresh) tomatoes to complete the broth. Continue to cook until the soup reaches a slow boil.

Add black beans. If using soaked black beans, simmer the soup longer to ensure the beans are cooked through and tender.

Add minced fresh herbs to the soup last, then salt and pepper to taste.

Elbow macaroni: In a separate pot, boil and drain noodles according to directions. Set noodles aside. If using gluten-free noodles they will swell and fall apart if left in the soup, so store noodles in a separate container for leftovers.

When serving, add ½ cup noodles into bowls, then ladle soup over.

Side suggestions: Toast GF bread and top with garlic butter, hummus, or melted cheese.

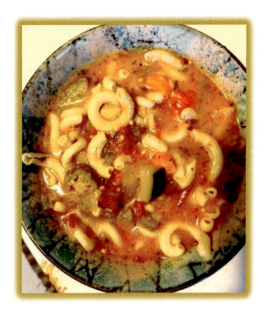

Pictured: Summer minestrone variation with squash, okra, carrots, and fresh diced tomatoes.

RECIPES FOR WINTER

French Lentil Soup with Roasted Potatoes

2–3 cups dry French (black) lentils
2–3 large cloves crushed garlic
1 large onion, chopped
3 medium carrots cut into rounds
2 Tbsp red wine
2 Tbsp balsamic vinegar
1 Tbsp sage
2 Tbsp olive oil
¼ cup nutritional yeast
6–8 cups water
salt and pepper to taste

DIRECTIONS

Start with a large pot and olive oil on medium heat.

Sauté garlic, onion, and carrot until they just begin to stick to the bottom.

Deglaze the pan by adding red wine and balsamic vinegar, then stir vigorously to lift the residue from the bottom of the pot (this gives the soup a hearty flavor).

Add lentils and water.

Stir in sage and nutritional yeast.

Simmer on low until lentils are soft (about 1–2 hours).

Roasted Potatoes

Cut potatoes into small chunks (keep skins on) and roll in freshly chopped rosemary, sea salt, and olive oil. Roast in 450° F oven for about 15 minutes. Flip them with a spatula and then cook an additional 15 minutes or until potatoes are tender and browned. Serve on side with the soup.

Black Bean Soup
with Cheesy Quesadillas

4 cups dry black beans (soaked overnight)
  or **3 cans precooked black beans**
1 qt jar canned tomatoes (from last summer,
  or 5–6 large tomatoes if in season)
2 large red and green peppers, diced (if in season)
  or 1 12 oz jar canned salsa (from last season or the store)
3 large cloves of garlic
⅓ cup Old Bay Seasoning
6 cups water
salt to taste

DIRECTIONS

Add to large pot black beans, tomatoes, peppers or salsa, garlic, and Old Bay Seasoning. Cook on medium-high heat, stirring continually until steam starts to rise and liquid is bubbling.

Add water, wait until it nears a boil, then turn heat down to low. Simmer about 60 minutes. If you used presoaked dry beans instead of canned, ensure the beans are tender. Salt to taste.

Cheesy Quesadillas

In a fry pan on low-medium heat add a drizzle of oil and place tortillas. Sprinkle shredded cheddar cheese on tortillas and fold in half. Cook until cheese is melted. If making several servings, transfer the quesadillas as they are made to a cookie sheet in a warm oven until served.

Vegan version: Omit cheese and dip fried/warmed tortillas in salsa.

RECIPES FOR WINTER

Kale-Garlic-Shiitake Soup with Carrot-Beet Ginger Salad

This garlic-rich mushroom soup is great for heart health and boosting the immune system.

- ½ **cup wheat berries** (presoaked overnight)
  or **1 cup brown rice** (cooked)
- **2 Tbsp olive oil**
- **1 cup or more thinly sliced shiitake mushrooms**
- **10 cloves of garlic**
- **¼ cup rice vinegar**
- **4 cups vegetable broth or water**
- **1 large bunch of kale, coarsely chopped**

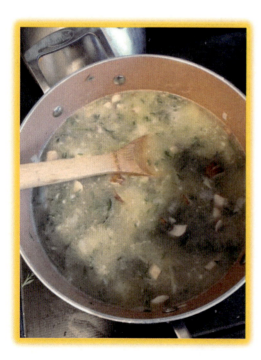

DIRECTIONS

Heat the olive oil in a large saucepan on medium heat, then add mushrooms. Sauté for about 10 minutes or until they start to brown.

Add crushed garlic and sauté a minute or two more.

Stir in vinegar, simmer until vinegar is almost evaporated, and deglaze the pan by scraping the bottom to lift up the brown bits.

Add wheat berries (or brown rice) along with vegetable broth or water. Bring to a boil, then reduce heat to simmer for 20 minutes.

Add kale and cook 10–20 more minutes until kale is tender.

RECIPES FOR WINTER

Carrot-Beet-Ginger Salad

> **3 carrots**
> **2 beets**
> **½ cup pine nuts**
>   ***or* pecan pieces**
> **1 Tbsp ginger**

DIRECTIONS

Shred root ingredients into salad bowl, toss with tahini dressing (below), top with nuts. Serve with soup.

Ginger Sesame Tahini Dressing

> **½ cup olive oil**
> **1 Tbsp ground ginger**
> **¼ balsamic vinegar**
> **1 Tbsp sesame oil**
> **2 Tbsp tahini**

Stir to blend, salting to taste.

This is one of Nitya's favorite salad dressings!

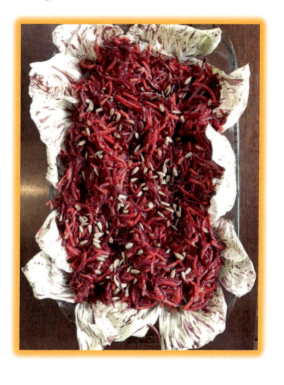

RECIPES FOR WINTER

Layered No-Noodle Veggie Lasagna

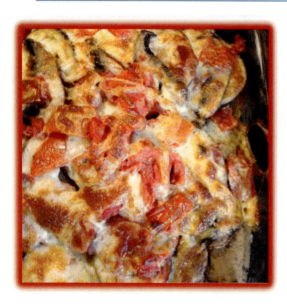

4–6 potatoes
1 large onion
2 Tbsp olive oil (to grease casserole dish)
1 large sweet potato (optional)
3–4 large portabella mushrooms
1 eggplant
1 qt jar canned tomatoes (from last summer)
smoked mozzarella
herbs (to taste):
    fresh dried basil, rosemary, oregano
salt and pepper to taste

DIRECTIONS

This is super-easy to make and so delicious!

Preheat oven to 425–450° F. Rub olive oil around the inside of a large casserole dish.

Thinly slice potatoes, onions, eggplant, mushrooms (also a sweet potato, if you like).

Like lasagna, begin layering ingredients until casserole dish is piled high (don't worry, it will cook down). Pour on top the canned tomatoes and sprinkle on herbs, along with a little salt and pepper.

Cover with aluminum foil and cook for approximately 30–40 minutes.

Remove aluminum foil, reduce heat to 350° F. Add sliced smoked mozzarella, then continue to bake uncovered for an additional 15–20 minutes. Watch to avoid charring the cheese.

Allow to sit for about 10 minutes before serving.

Recipes for Winter

Spaghetti Squash & Cheese with a Side of Steamed Greens

1 large spaghetti squash
Parmesan cheese (optional)
1 Tbsp olive oil (for pan)
1–2 cloves garlic, crushed
small jar of tomato sauce (from last summer)
bunch of kale, chard or spinach
¼ cup roasted sunflower or pumpkin seeds

DIRECTIONS

Preheat oven to 400° F.

Cut spaghetti squash in half lengthwise and scoop out the seeds. Place *face-down* on oiled, shallow baking pan. Bake for about 40 minutes.

Just before the squash is done, heat tomato sauce in saucepan on low-medium heat. Add crushed garlic and salt to taste.

Then in a steamer with boiling water, add greens, cover and cook for a minute or two—*do not overcook!*

Greens can also be enjoyed as a salad with dressing.

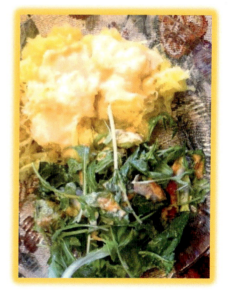

Carefully remove squash from pan and flip over onto a plate (use oven mitts to ensure you don't burn fingers). With a fork, scrape the stringy squash meats out into a medium-sized serving bowl.

Serve squash and top with tomato sauce and add grated Parmesan, if desired. Add steamed greens or salad on the side and sprinkle with seeds.

Note: This is a flexible meal that can be adjusted in many ways. Pictured above is spaghetti squash without sauce, and with a raw greens salad.

RECIPES FOR WINTER

Roasted Root Medley
with Goat Cheese & Pine Nuts

4 beets
4–6 medium potatoes
2 sweet potatoes
4 large carrots
1 large onion
container of local goat cheese (optional)
½ cup olive oil
½ tsp sea salt
2 Tbsp fresh rosemary, minced
½ cup pine nuts
  or **roasted pumpkin seeds**
  or **pecan or walnut pieces**

DIRECTIONS

Preheat oven to 450° F.

Cube the root veggies, but slice onion in large wedges.

Mix sea salt and crushed rosemary into the olive oil.

Put roots in casserole dish and toss with olive oil mixture, coating veggies thoroughly. Sprinkle nuts on top.

Bake uncovered for about 45 minutes or until the veggies are tender when poked with a fork.

Remove from oven and toss in local goat cheese, if desired.

Serve with a side of steamed local greens—chard, kale, or spinach.

Creamy Carrot Ginger Soup

3–4 medium to large carrots sliced
1 large sweet potato
1 Tbsp olive oil
1 large clove of garlic
2–3 Tbsp minced fresh ginger
1 Tbsp turmeric
½ cup nutritional yeast
1–2 Tbsp apple cider vinegar
4–6 cups of water

DIRECTIONS

Add olive oil to large pot on medium heat. When hot, add veggies and simmer for about 5 minutes.

Pour in water and simmer until veggies are soft.

In a saucepan add ginger, garlic, and vinegar and simmer on low. Add nutritional yeast and turmeric, stirring as you add ingredients. Set aside.

Puree veggies using a hand mixer (if using a blender, return to pot), then add contents from saucepan.

Simmer for about 30 minutes to assimilate the flavors.

Serve with a kale and arugula salad with ginger tahini dressing (page 9).

Variation: For a spicy kick, top your bowl of soup with hot sauce.

RECIPES FOR WINTER

Thai Peanut Noodles with Steamed Chard

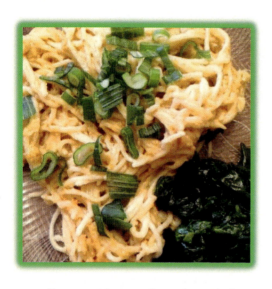

1 pkg of rice spaghetti noodles
1 cup fresh peanut butter
¼ cup Bragg's Liquid Aminos
   or **soy sauce**
2 Tbsp sesame oil
¼ cup rice vinegar
2 green chilis or chives

DIRECTIONS

Cook noodles according to package directions, drain. Do not overcook.

In a medium saucepan over medium heat, stirring with a wooden spoon, add the sesame oil, peanut butter, Bragg's, and vinegar. Continue to stir until the peanut butter softens and blends with other ingredients.

Add enough water to make it sauce-like and stir until smooth. About 1 cup of water should be enough.

Put the cooked pasta back in the pot and stir in the peanut sauce with a large cooking fork to coat the noodles but not turn it into mush (which can happen if using a spoon).

Serve on plates and top with sliced chili peppers or chives.

One of my daughter's favorite meals!

Steamed Chard

| **1 bunch chard** | **fresh ground garlic** | **salt or tahini** |

Steam washed greens 1–2 minutes (until just cooked). Season to taste.

Recipes for Winter

Scalloped Potatoes with Steamed Greens

6 large potatoes
½ cup organic salted butter
½ cup gluten-free flour
3½ cups water
2 Tbsp Bragg's Liquid Aminos *or* soy sauce
1 tsp garlic powder
½ tsp turmeric
¼ cup veggie oil
¼ cup nutritional yeast

DIRECTIONS

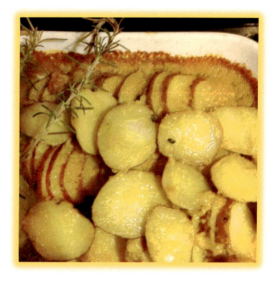

Preheat Oven to 450° F.

Slice potatoes thin and spread in lightly butter-greased dish.

Bring water to boil in a pot.

In a medium saucepan whisk together the flour and butter over a low heat until melted and thickened.

Stir remaining ingredients into saucepan, then *gradually* add boiling water, stirring briskly for a few minutes or until the sauce is smooth and thick.

Pour sauce over the potatoes, ensuring they are thoroughly covered.

Cover dish with aluminum foil and bake for 30 minutes, then cool for 10.

Serve with steamed greens on the side (see previous recipe).

This is total comfort food! Leftovers are fabulous!

Note: I often use this sauce as a gravy during the holidays.

RECIPES FOR WINTER

Winter Root Soup

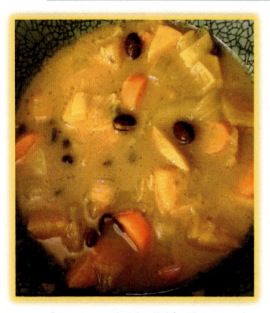

3–4 medium carrots
1 large sweet potato
2 beets with greens
1½ cups local mushrooms
2 large cloves of garlic
1 Tbsp olive oil
½ cup nutritional yeast
1 Tbsp turmeric
1 tsp (or more) rosemary
1 tsp (or more) thyme
1 can organic black beans

DIRECTIONS

Slice carrots into half-inch segments. Cube the beets and sweet potato (set aside greens for steamed side dish). Chop mushrooms.

In a large pot on medium heat, add olive oil. When hot, add root veggies and mushrooms. Sauté for 20 minutes, stirring occasionally.

Add the black beans, garlic, turmeric, rosemary and thyme, then simmer another 10 minutes.

Add 6 cups of water along with the nutritional yeast. Return to boil, reduce heat to low, cover and simmer 10 minutes, stirring occasionally.

Salt and pepper to taste.

Steam beet greens for a few minutes until just wilted for a side or to top your bowl of soup.

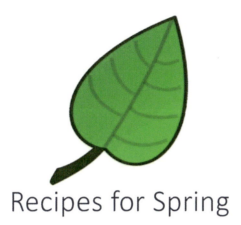

Recipes for Spring

Asparagus with Garlic Pasta

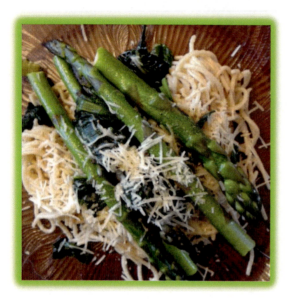

A delightfully light dinner that is quick and easy to make.

1 bunch local asparagus
1 package rice pasta
2 cloves garlic
⅓ cup olive oil
Parmesan cheese (optional)

DIRECTIONS

Pasta: Boil pasta according to directions. While pasta is boiling, begin asparagus to ensure everything will be ready at the same time.

Turn off heat. Drain pasta and return to pot. In a small mixing bowl, combine olive oil, crushed garlic, and a pinch of salt. Pour over pasta and toss.

Asparagus: To prepare the asparagus, snap the stalks so they break, discarding the bottom third, keeping the more tender upper portions.

In a saucepan with a half inch of boiling water add asparagus, cover and steam for 2–3 minutes. *Do not overcook*—they should be bendy when lifted, not floppy and falling apart.

Serve pasta with several stalks of asparagus on top, sprinkled with Parmesan (optional) to finish.

Tip: Asparagus arrives at the farmers' markets in April and is only around for a couple of months. When buying asparagus look for the thinner stalks. Thick ones tend to be somewhat fibrous and woody.

Variation: I sometimes like to steam some spinach to toss *into* the pasta for an extra-nourishing entree.

RECIPES FOR SPRING

Indian Chickpea Curry on Rice

2 cups rice (to make 4 cups cooked rice)
1 can of chickpeas, drained
3 medium carrots
2–4 medium potatoes
1 medium onion
½-inch piece of ginger minced
1 Tbsp curry powder
¼ tsp cumin
1 tsp turmeric
2 Tbsp peanut oil or sunflower oil

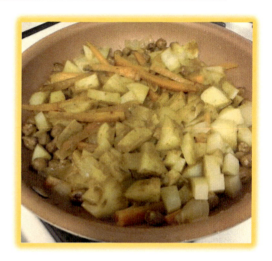

DIRECTIONS

Start rice (add to 4 cups boiling water, cover, reduce heat to medium-low, remove from heat after 30 minutes).

Slice carrot into medallions or julienne. Slice onion into thick wedges and then halve them. Cube potatoes. Sauté these ingredients in peanut oil on medium-high heat for three minutes, stirring frequently.

Reduce heat to medium, then add minced ginger and spices. Stir to blend for three more minutes.

Stir in chickpeas and about 1½ cups water. Cover and simmer on low heat 20 minutes.

Serve on rice with a side of steamed asparagus or roasted Brussels sprouts (see 53).

Salt and Pepper to taste.

Optional: Add a little Asian chili relish for a fiery kick.

RECIPES FOR SPRING

Spring Greens Salad with Quinoa

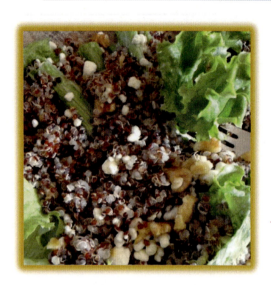

1–2 cups prepared red quinoa
local arugula
local mixed spring greens
local carrots, grated
½ grapefruit
½ cup walnuts
½ cup local goat cheese
  (optional)

DIRECTIONS

Fill a large salad bowl with washed leafy ingredients.

Cube grapefruit. Grate carrots.

Add these ingredients to the greens and toss until well mixed. Next, toss in quinoa, walnuts and goat cheese.

Add enough of the dressing to wet the leaves and flavor the quinoa. See dressing recipe on next page.

Note: Since this one dish is a full meal, consider that the portion size is a dinner plate heaping with salad. It is one of my favorite warm weather meals because it feels so light and healthy.

RECIPES FOR SPRING

♥ Miss Nitya's Yoga Camp Salad Dressing

⅔ cup olive oil
½ cup red wine vinegar
2 Tbsp tahini
1 Tbsp local honey
salt to taste

DIRECTIONS

Combine all ingredients in a bowl.

Stir thoroughly with a fork until ingredients are well blended.

Variations: As good as this dressing is using the instructions above, this recipe is essentially a base from which you can come up with your own favorite variations. Let the following ideas inspire you (some of which may require a blender).

- Add 1 pureed carrot for a textured sweetness.
- Add ¼ cup of fresh ground almond butter–adding enough water to thin to the right consistency
- Blend in a clove of garlic and/or a Tbsp of one or two fresh herbs (such as thyme, rosemary, sage, lavender, basil, mustard seed, coriander, dill, chives), to enhance flavor.
- For an Asian kick try grated ginger and/or a tsp of Bragg's Liquid Aminos (or soy sauce), maybe even a ½ tsp of horseradish.
- Try substituting the vinegar with lemon juice, or another vinegar, such as balsamic or Bragg's Apple Cider Vinegar.
- Tang it up with a Tbsp of fresh-squeezed orange juice (or orange zest), or make it succulent with half of a peach, pureed.
- Add strawberries (as I did on page 23) for a sweet-tart twist!

RECIPES FOR SPRING

Sweet Potato and Black Bean Chili

1 large sweet potato, peeled and diced
1 large onion
4 cloves garlic, crushed
2 Tbsp olive oil
2 Tbsp chili powder
2 tsp cumin
2½ cups water
2 cans of organic black beans
1 jar of salsa or tomatoes
   (put up from last summer)
½ cup fresh local cilantro

DIRECTIONS

Heat oil in large pot over medium-high heat. Add sweet potato and onion, stirring often for about 5 minutes.

Add garlic, chili powder, cumin, and salt to taste. Mix well.

Add water and bring to a simmer.

Cover and cook on low heat for about 20–30 minutes, or until sweet potatoes are tender.

Add beans, tomatoes or salsa, and turn heat to medium high, stirring often for a few minutes until simmering resumes.

Reduce heat and allow to simmer another 5 minutes.

Serve topped with fresh cilantro.

RECIPES FOR SPRING

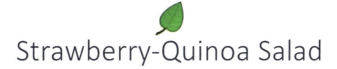

Strawberry-Quinoa Salad

This is a super quick and nutritious lunch or light dinner for a warm spring day.

> local spinach, washed and de-stemmed
> local fresh salad greens
> ½ cup roasted sunflower seeds
> 6–12 local strawberries, sliced (tops removed)
> 1 cup cooked and cooled quinoa

Mix all ingredients in a large bowl. Toss in the dressing (see below).

Note: Adjust quantities as needed depending on the number of servings required. Each serving should fill a large dinner plate. I would likely use 2 cups spring greens and 4 cups spinach to feed a family of four.

Miss Nitya's
Yoga Camp Strawberry *Salad Dressing*

> 1 cup olive oil   ½ cup red wine vinegar
> 2 Tbsp tahini   1 Tbsp local honey
> 4–6 local strawberries   salt to taste

Use a mixer to blend ingredients thoroughly until smooth.

RECIPES FOR SPRING

Chana Masala Stuffed Sweet Potatoes

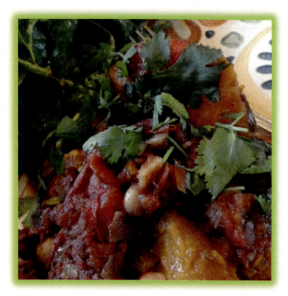

4 medium sweet potatoes
1½ Tbsp coconut oil
1 medium local onion
2 cloves garlic, minced
2–3 tsp fresh ginger root, minced
1–2 Tbsp garam masala
2 tsp paprika
salt and pepper to taste
1 cup roasted tomatoes (frozen from last summer)
1 medium jar of canned tomatoes (put up from last summer)
1 can cooked chickpeas
1 cup full-fat coconut milk
1 small bunch fresh, local cilantro, minced

DIRECTIONS

Preheat oven to 425° F.

Scrub, rinse, then prick the sweet potatoes several times with a fork and place on a baking sheet. Roast for about 45 minutes or until tender.

While the sweet potatoes bake, add coconut oil to a large pan over medium-high heat. Dice onions and stir into oil; cook until slightly soft.

Add the garlic, ginger, garam masala, paprika, salt and pepper; cook for about 1 more minute, stirring often.

Add the roasted tomatoes, canned tomatoes and chickpeas. Bring to a boil, then reduce heat and simmer for 20 minutes; stir occasionally.

Pour in the coconut milk and continue to simmer for 5 minutes more. Taste and adjust seasonings if needed.

RECIPES FOR SPRING

Slice open sweet potatoes lengthwise (cutting deep along the top), then scoop a healthy portion of the chana masala filling into each.

Garnish with the minced cilantro.

Note: This recipe produces four large servings. For more people, increase the number of sweet potatoes and other ingredients accordingly. For eight half-sized servings, prepare this same recipe, but pile the topping onto individual sweet potato halves.

RECIPES FOR SPRING

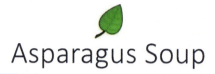

Asparagus Soup

MODIFIED FROM A RECIPE BY MISS NITYA'S MOM, BEA GRIFFITH

2 cups sliced leeks
3 Tbsp butter
2–3 Tbsp gluten-free flour
3–4 cups water
½ cup nutritional yeast
2 cups cubed potatoes
1 carrot, sliced
1 stalk celery, sliced
1 bunch local asparagus, chopped in pieces
fresh, local dill
salt and pepper to taste
1 clove garlic, crushed
1 cup organic heavy cream (optional)

DIRECTIONS

Sauté leeks in butter for about 10 minutes on low heat until soft.

Add GF flour, water, and nutritional yeast, then mix well.

Then add potatoes, carrot, celery, asparagus (keep tips out and set aside), dill, garlic, and salt/pepper. Let simmer for about 20 minutes or until veggies are tender.

Puree with a hand mixer or in a blender, add cream and blend until smooth.

Can be served hot or chilled. Garnish with asparagus tips.

Serve with a side salad (see page 36).

RECIPES FOR SPRING

Chesapeake Bay Potato-Leek Soup

6 medium potatoes, cut in chunks
1 bunch of local leeks
½ cup nutritional yeast
2 heaping Tbsp Old Bay Seasoning
4–6 cups water
2 cloves garlic, crushed

DIRECTIONS

In a large pot add olive oil, crushed garlic, and sliced leeks. Simmer on low-medium heat until garlic is browning and leeks are softening.

Add water, nutritional yeast, potatoes, and Old Bay, stirring over medium heat until simmering at a low boil.

Reduce heat back to low and simmer covered for 20–30 minutes or until potatoes are tender.

Use a hand mixer to cream the soup, leaving it just chunky enough to be interesting.

Garnish with a sprinkle of Old Bay.

Note: Can be served hot or chilled.

Tip: Serve with local crusty bread and a side of steamed spinach, kale, or chard.

RECIPES FOR SPRING

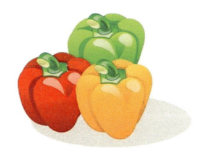

Recipes for Summer

RECIPES FOR SUMMER

Crabby Cakes with Sliced Heirloom Tomatoes and Potato Salad

Having grown up in the city of Baltimore and the Eastern Shore of Maryland, crab was a regular part of my summer menu until I became a vegetarian. Luckily, these crabby cakes are so close to the real thing that some may not even notice. (Freeze up shredded zucchini every summer to enjoy these in the wintertime, too).

Tip: I often triple this recipe to have ample leftovers.

- **2 cups or more coarsely shredded zucchini**
  (easiest to do in a food processor)
- **1 cup GF breadcrumbs**
- **1 farm-fresh egg, beaten**
- **1–2 Tbsp or more of Old Bay Seasoning**
- **1 tsp Dijon mustard**
- **1 Tbsp mayonnaise or Vegannaise**
  (Duke's is local to Richmond, Virginia)
- **oil for frying** (not butter or olive, as they scorch easily)
- **salt to taste**

DIRECTIONS

Place grated zucchini in a sieve and sprinkle with a little salt (this is to aid water extraction but go easy so as not to make the zucchini taste salty), let sit for 30 minutes. Squeeze to drain excess liquid.

In a large bowl, mix breadcrumbs and zucchini together.

Place beaten egg, Old Bay, Dijon, and mayo in a medium-size bowl and mix well, then pour into the zucchini-bread crumb mixture. Mix gently, then let sit for about 10 minutes.

Form into patties (about eight 4-inch patties or twelve 3-inch patties).

Heat oil in a pan until medium hot (not smoking), then fry up the cakes until they're lightly browned on each side. Set cooked patties on paper towel to absorb excess oils.

Note: Great topped with wasabi mayonnaise. Serve with sliced local tomatoes and potato salad.

Variation: A friend has also made these with one grated medium potato and a Tbsp of nutritional yeast mixed in with the zucchini and bread-crumbs with good results.

Potato Salad

8–10 medium local potatoes
1 Tbsp Dijon mustard
1 small (or ½ large) onion, diced

¼–½ cup mayonnaise
2 tsp red wine vinegar
fresh dill

Cut potatoes into large bite-sized chunks, then boil until tender.

Mix well cooked potatoes with onion, Dijon, mayo, and vinegar.

Garnish with fresh dill.

Option: 2 Tbsp of local relish in the mix is a nice variation.

Recipes for Summer

Fried Okra on Pasta with Tomato Sauce

Okra is a hardy plant that takes up little space in your garden but can grow to 7 feet. It will yield into early autumn. Pick okra when pods are 3 to 4 inches long (if allowed to grow too big they become fibrous and tough). There are many things you can do with them—batter frying for a tasty side or snack, boiling for gumbo or minestrone soup, pickling, and this fabulous pasta dish.

12 or more medium-sized okra
cooking oil
2 farm-fresh eggs
2 cups gluten-free flour
2 Tbsp blended Italian herbs (fresh is best)
4 large tomatoes
2 cloves garlic
1 package gluten-free pasta
shredded Parmesan (optional)

DIRECTIONS

Puree tomatoes until smooth.

In one bowl mix flour with Italian herbs. In another bowl beat the eggs (vegan option: replace eggs with 2 Tbsp potato flour well beaten into ¼ cup of water).

In a large skillet heat oil on medium high heat.

Drop okra in egg batter then roll into flour mixture.

Carefully place into hot oil and cook until golden, stirring occasionally.

Cook GF pasta according to package directions. Drain and return to pot.

Pour the tomato sauce over the pasta, then squeeze 2 cloves of garlic through a press, and toss lightly.

Serve pasta with okra on top and sprinkle with Parmesan cheese.

Recipes for Summer

Loaded Salad with Lentils

To judge the amount of ingredients for a large salad for family and/or guests, I choose a salad bowl large enough for everyone, then fill it half-way with local field greens and arugula, then add to it whatever I have in the fridge or garden.

Serves 2–3 people

- **2 cups lentils**
- **field greens and arugula, to half-fill large bowl**
- **½ cucumber, sliced thinly**
- **1 large heirloom tomato, cubed**
- **1 yellow squash, cubed**
- **1 red, yellow or green pepper, thinly sliced**
- **¼ of a large onion, sliced**
- **8 raw okra, sliced**
- **¼ cup raw or roasted sunflower seeds**
- **Miss Nitya's Yoga Camp Salad Dressing** (page 21)

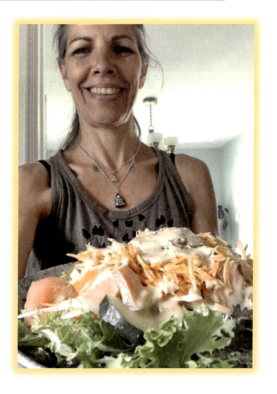

DIRECTIONS

In a medium saucepan add 2 cups of black lentils and cover with water. Bring to a boil and then simmer for 20–30 minutes, until lentils are tender). Cool lentils and then spoon about 1 cup onto the salad.

Toss all the salad ingredients together with the dressing.

Tip: Be creative! Try different veggies.

RECIPES FOR SUMMER

Noodles with Summer Veggies in a Thai Peanut Sauce

If your local store doesn't carry them, buy cellophane rice noodles from an Asian market.

- **1 pkg cellophane rice noodles** (4–6 servings)
- **1 medium zucchini**
- **2 medium summer yellow squash**
- **1–2 small eggplants, Ichiban if available**
- **1 medium onion**

Thai Peanut Sauce

- **2 cloves garlic, minced**
- **1 Tbsp fresh ginger, minced**
- **2 tsp sesame oil**
- **½ cup unsalted peanuts** (whole or crushed)
- **3 tsp rice vinegar**
- **½ cup of Bragg's or Soy Sauce**
- **½ cup of fresh ground peanut butter**
- **1 cup of water**
- **1 minced hot chili pepper** (optional)

DIRECTIONS

In a large skillet add a little vegetable oil and sauté sliced veggies until tender. Set veggies aside on a plate.

Begin heating water for the noodles in a separate pot.

In the same skillet used for the veggies, begin making the sauce by heating the sesame oil, then adding the minced garlic and ginger, allowing a minute to infuse the oil.

Next, stir in the other sauce ingredients. Set heat to low and continue stirring until well-mixed. Add the veggies and continue to sauté for a few minutes.

RECIPES FOR SUMMER

When the pot of water is at a rolling boil, add noodles and cook for duration indicated on package (these cook fast, so watch carefully to prevent overcooking).

Drain noodles, rinse in cold water. Serve pasta on plates with sauced veggies spooned on top.

RECIPES FOR SUMMER

Stuffed Red Peppers with Side Salad

---

4 large red peppers (1 per person)
2 cups prepared brown rice or quinoa
1 medium onion, diced
1 cup corn *off* **the cob**
1 large tomato, diced
4–6 leaves of fresh basil, cut fine
Local goat cheese (optional)

DIRECTIONS

Prepare rice or quinoa.

Preheat oven to 375° F.

Toss the diced onion, tomato, basil, and corn in the rice.

Salt to taste.

Cut the tops off the peppers and scoop out the seeds. (I love to save seeds to dry and plant next summer.)

Scoop the rice veggie mixture into each pepper until nearly full. If desired, sprinkle goat cheese on top of each pepper.

Put peppers on a lightly oiled cook pan and place in oven for about 30 minutes. Check periodically for progress.

Pepper should be tender enough to easily cut.

Side Salad

Cut 2 or 3 large, local, heirloom tomatoes into wedges. Sprinkle with minced fresh basil and balsamic vinegar. Lightly salt and pepper, if desired.

RECIPES FOR SUMMER

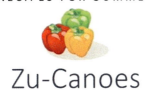

Zu-Canoes

My daughter Bea and I would have a cooking day once a week. Here she is filling the Zu-Canoes before baking. It was so much fun, educational, and delicious too! She has continued experimenting in the kitchen into adulthood.

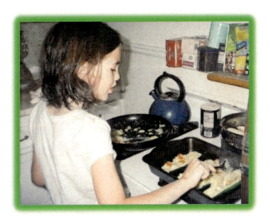

- **6–8 medium small zucchinis**
  (2 Zu-Canoes per person)
- **2 cups prepared quinoa or Brown Rice**
- **1 medium onion**
- **1 red pepper**
- **1 green pepper**
- **1 large tomato, diced**
- **4–6 leaves fresh basil, cut fine**
- **grated Parmesan or local cheese** (optional)

DIRECTIONS

Prepare quinoa or rice. Preheat Oven to 375° F.

Dice the onion, tomato, peppers, and basil, then sauté over medium heat in a saucepan with a little olive oil until veggies are tender and soft.

Mix the quinoa or rice in with the veggies. Salt to taste.

Slice the zucchinis lengthwise and scoop out the seeds, leaving enough room to add filling.

Scoop the veggie mixture into each zucchini until more than full, then top with grated cheese (if desired) before baking.

Put Zu-canoes on a greased cookie sheet and bake about 30 minutes, checking periodically to make sure cheese doesn't scorch. Zu-canoes should be tender enough to cut with ease when done.

Serve with Side Salad (see previous page).

RECIPES FOR SUMMER

Gumbo with Sweet Cucumber Salad

12 or more sliced okra
6 med-large heirloom tomatoes
1 red pepper
1 medium zucchini
1 medium yellow squash
1 Tbsp Old Bay Seasoning
2 cloves minced garlic
2 ears of corn

1 pint green beans
2 green peppers
1½ cups uncooked brown rice
1 Tbsp cumin
1 Tbsp chili powder
1 large onion
salt and pepper to taste
chili peppers for heat (optional)

DIRECTIONS

Slice and cube all the veggies. Cut kernels from ears of corn.

Put about 1 Tbsp olive oil in large pot on medium heat and add the veggies. Stir occasionally until veggies begin to soften.

Add garlic and spices, stirring until well blended.

Add 4–6 cups of water and increase heat until gumbo starts to bubble.

Add uncooked rice, cover pot, reduce heat to simmer for about an hour, stirring occasionally. *(You could also cook the rice separately, then add to each bowl.)*

Sweet Cucumber Salad

2 medium cucumbers, sliced thin
1 tsp agave or maple syrup
2–3 sprigs of fresh dill, chopped

½ cup balsamic vinegar
¼ red onion diced fine
pinch of salt (optional)

DIRECTIONS

In a medium sized bowl mix vinegar and sweetener, then adding the onion and dill. Salt conservatively (if desired).

Lay cucumber slices flat in bowl so they are marinating in the dressing for 30–60 minutes. If desired, chill in the refrigerator before serving.

RECIPES FOR SUMMER

Southwest Quinoa Salad

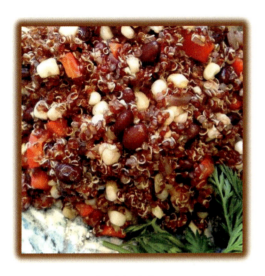

4 cups cooked quinoa
½ red onion, diced
2 ears of corn
¼ cup fresh cilantro, minced
2 bell peppers, diced
   (1 yellow, 1 orange or red)
1 can organic black beans
1 large ripe avocado, cubed
feta cheese chunks (optional)

DIRECTIONS

Cut corn off cobs and put in a bowl along with the diced onion, cilantro, and pepper.

Toss in the black beans, cooked quinoa, and feta (optional) until thoroughly mixed.

Dressing

½ cup olive oil
¼ cup balsamic vinegar
1 cup cantaloupe, cubed
1 tsp local honey
salt to taste

DIRECTIONS

Blend dressing ingredients with a mixer until smooth.

Pour onto Southwest Quinoa Salad and toss well.

RECIPES FOR SUMMER

♥Sesame Noodles with Squash and a Tomato Basil Salad

This is a really simple meal that the camp kids adore!

- 1 pkg GF pasta, cooked
- ½ cup sesame oil
- ¼ cup sesame seeds
- 1 Tbsp rice vinegar
- 2 Tbsp Bragg's Liquid Aminos *or* soy sauce
- 4 medium yellow squash
- 2 medium zucchinis

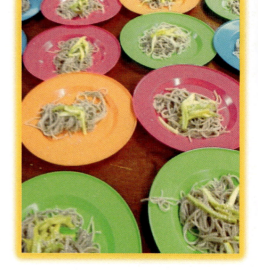

DIRECTIONS

Toss *cooked* pasta in a large pot with sesame oil until well coated.

Cut squash and zucchini julienne style (long thin strips) and place in a hot saucepan with a little cooking oil to sauté. Add Bragg's Liquid Aminos and rice vinegar then simmer until well cooked.

Now turn pasta pot on a low heat (just to warm) and add squash along with any leftover liquid. Toss to avoid sticking to the pan while heating.

Serve pasta with sesame seeds sprinkled on top.

Salt to taste.

Tomato Basil Salad

Serve fresh tomato slices and top with whole basil leaves, the drizzle with balsamic vinegar and half as much honey.

Variations: The salad can also be presented as cubed tomatoes and torn-up basil leaves tossed in dressing. Either option can also be served on a bed of greens, if preferred.

RECIPES FOR SUMMER

♥Summer Veggie Soup with side of Roasted Potatoes

2 Tbsp olive oil
10–12 large tomatoes
4 cloves of garlic, minced
2 medium zucchinis, chopped
2–3 yellow squash, chopped
1 large onion, sliced
salt to taste

1 cup shelled peas
1 pint basket of green beans
kernels from 4 ears corn
¼ cup balsamic vinegar
¼ to ⅓ cup minced fresh herbs
 (basil, thyme, rosemary
 and/or oregano)

DIRECTIONS

In a large pot simmer garlic and sliced onion in olive oil on medium-high heat. As the garlic and onion begin to brown, add the vinegar.

Using a wooden spoon, vigorously lift the browned garlic and onion residue from the bottom of the pot (this is called deglazing and makes for a richer broth). Turn heat to medium-low.

Add the chopped zucchinis, squash, peas, green beans, and corn to the pot.

Puree tomatoes with a mixer, then pour into the pot along with about 4–6 cups of water.

Add minced herbs to the soup, then salt to taste.

Allow to simmer for at least an hour.

Roasted Potatoes

Preheat oven to 450° F.

Quarter-cut 1 quart of small red-skinned potatoes. Toss in olive oil and sea salt with Old Bay Seasoning until lightly coated.

Roast in the oven for about 30 minutes or until browned and tender.

Recipes for Summer

♥ Thai Noodles with Peanut Sauce

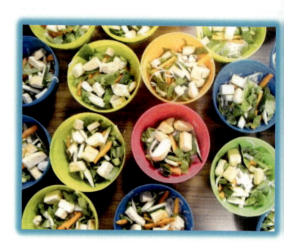

1 block Twin Oaks tofu
   (local GMO-free)
4 medium carrots
1 cucumber
salad greens
1 bok choy
¼ cup cilantro, minced
**½ pkg Asian cellophane rice
   noodles** (for 4–5 servings)

DIRECTIONS

Cube tofu (you can opt to fry the tofu in oil or use it raw).

Julienne cut cucumber and carrot (long, thin strips).

Slice bok choy thinly from base to the top leaves.

Cook noodles according to package directions. Transfer to colander and drain and rinse in cold water.

To serve, first place about 1 cup noodles in bottom of each bowl.

Next, add handful of salad greens, cilantro and bok choy.

Then top with cucumbers, carrots and tofu.

Peanut Sauce

2 Tbsp honey
1 Tbsp rice vinegar
½ cup HOT water
½ cup crushed unsalted peanuts

**2 Tbsp Bragg's Liquid Aminos
   or soy sauce**
1 tsp garlic chili sauce
   (caution: very spicy)

DIRECTIONS

Whisk liquid dressing ingredients with a fork and drizzle over each bowl. Sprinkle crushed peanuts on top. Season with additional Bragg's or soy sauce, if desired.

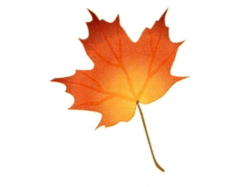

Recipes for Autumn

RECIPES FOR AUTUMN

Greek Casserole

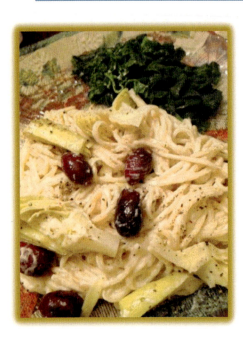

1 pkg GF pasta *or* **4 cups cooked rice**

1 small jar marinated roasted artichoke hearts

1 can northern or garbanzo beans

1 small jar Kalamata olives, pitted, drained

½ cup olive oil

2 cloves garlic, minced

feta cheese (optional)

seasonal greens (kale, spinach or chard— either blended in the casserole or served on the side, as shown in picture)

DIRECTIONS

Prepare pasta (or rice) and put in a large pot.

Pour olive oil and garlic in and toss to coat.

Separate leaves of artichoke hearts and allow *some* of the oils from the artichoke jar to go in as well.

Slice ½ the jar of olives and add along with the beans.

Serve with feta crumbled on top and steamed greens.

RECIPES FOR AUTUMN

Italian Fried Eggplant

1 large eggplant sliced ¼ inch thick
2 cups gluten-free flour
¼ cup oregano, thyme and basil, minced
2 farm-fresh eggs, beaten
6–8 large tomatoes, pureed
2 cloves of garlic
frying oil
1 pkg of gluten-free pasta (Bombolini pasta made in Richmond is amazing!)
fresh grated Parmesan cheese (optional)

DIRECTIONS

In a large skillet heat oil on medium heat until popping.

Prepare 2 bowls for dipping: one with the beaten eggs and one with the flour mixed with ½ the herb blend.

Dip eggplant slices into the egg batter and then toss to cover in flour. Place carefully in frying pan. Ensure heat is not too hot.

Line a baking sheet with folded paper towels and place in open oven on low heat (around 200° F). As each eggplant slice finishes frying, place on this tray to draw off excess oil and to keep warm.

Prepare pasta according to package directions. Drain and set aside.

Tomato Sauce: In a medium pot on medium heat, pour in the pureed tomato, crushed garlic, and the rest of the minced herbs. Salt to taste. Heat until very warm, stirring occasionally.

Serve cooked pasta on the plates, place 2–3 fried eggplant slices on top, then ladle tomato sauce on top. Sprinkle generously Parmesan cheese to finish (optional).

RECIPES FOR AUTUMN

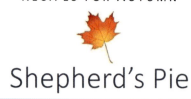

Shepherd's Pie

8–10 large potatoes
1 package of plant-based "sausage" (GMO-free), or a package of LightLife Smoky Tempeh, or leftover crumbled Grandma Mary Veggie Burger (see recipe page 72)
2 large red or yellow onions
2–3 cups roasted peppers
(frozen and put up from last summer)
aged cheddar cheese or vegan cheese (see recipe page 47)
1 stick organic salted butter

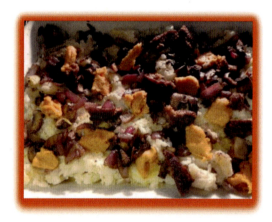

DIRECTIONS

Boil potatoes until cooked. Mash with masher or hand mixer while adding half of the butter (cut into pats). Blend until smooth mashed potatoes.

Preheat oven to 375° F. Butter a casserole dish and spread half of the potatoes in.

Slice the onions and "sausage", tempeh or veggie burger crumble. Then sauté those ingredients with peppers in a little olive oil on medium high heat until lightly browned.

Layer the veggies and meat substitute over the potatoes, then dollop the rest of the potatoes on top, spreading to cover.

Take chunks of cheddar cheese or vegan cheese along with the remaining butter and stick into this top layer of mashed potatoes.

Bake approximately 30–45 minutes or until top is golden, cheese melted, and entire casserole is hot.

A great winter holiday meal with steamed greens served on the side.

RECIPES FOR AUTUMN

Raw Vegan Cheddar Cheese

- 1½ cups raw cashews
  (presoaked overnight in water)
- 2 heaping Tbsp chopped sundried tomatoes (soaked with cashews)
- 1 heaping Tbsp white miso paste
- 1 Tbsp Bragg's Apple Cider Vinegar
- ½ tsp dry ground mustard powder
- ¼ cup nutritional yeast
- 1 tsp sea salt
- 1 tsp onion powder
- ½ tsp smoked paprika
- ¼ tsp turmeric
- ½ cup *refined* coconut oil
  (unrefined leaves aftertaste)

DIRECTIONS

Drain water from the soaking cashews and sundried tomatoes and rinse with fresh water. Drain well.

Put cashews and tomatoes in a food processor and blend until it forms a paste.

Add all the remaining ingredients except the coconut oil and blend thoroughly in processor.

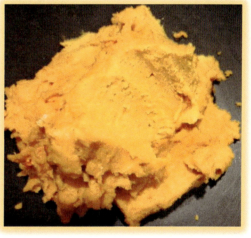

Add the coconut oil and continue blending 3–5 minutes until smooth.

Cover and refrigerate for at least four hours or until cheese is firm (overnight is preferable).

You can now form the cheese into a large ball, log, or brick for slicing. This makes a soft, delicious cheese!

Tip: For newbies who might be put-off by the phrase "vegan cheese," you can call this "Sundried Tomato-Cashew Pâté" and they'll devour it. Mindset is everything.

Options: For a festive touch, roll the cheese ball or log in toppings, such as slivered almonds, pecan pieces, or crushed fresh herbs like sage, black pepper, thyme, and/or rosemary.

RECIPES FOR AUTUMN

Asian Rice Noodle Stir Fry

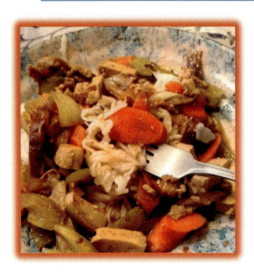

1 pkg Asian cellophane
   rice noodles
4 carrots, cut in chunks
1 medium onion, sliced
1½ cups sliced shiitake
   mushrooms*
bok choy, if available, sliced
1 block tofu, cubed
   (Twin Oaks is local to
   Virginia)
1 Tbsp sesame oil
2 inch chunk of fresh ginger
   root, minced
Bragg's Liquid Aminos
   or soy sauce

Tip: For mushrooms local to Richmond, Rudy's Exotic Mushrooms are sold at Ellwood Thompson's Natural Market.

DIRECTIONS

This is the easiest meal to put together—flavorful and nutritious.

Cook noodles according to package directions. Do not overcook! Briefly rinse cooked noodles in cool water to avoid them turning into paste.

Fry tofu in sesame oil on medium-high heat, turning every few minutes to brown slightly on both sides.

Add onion, ginger, carrot, and mushrooms until carrots begin to soften but are still firm.

Add bok choy (if using it) and continue to cook a few more minutes. Toss in noodles and season to taste with Bragg's Liquid Aminos or soy sauce.

RECIPES FOR AUTUMN

Fall Veggie Casserole

2–3 medium potatoes
2 medium zucchinis
   (if still available)
1 large onion
3–4 large carrots
1 large eggplant
3–4 red and/or green
   tomatoes
large ball of mozzarella
sea salt and fresh rosemary

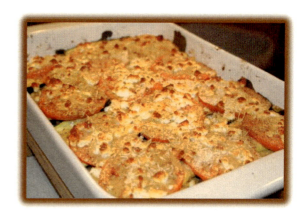

DIRECTIONS

Oil a large baking dish and preheat oven to 450° F.

Slice all of the vegetables and mozzarella to medium width slabs and layer in dish.

There should be 2 complete layers with the mozzarella on top. And yes, this may be taller than the dish, but it will settle down as it cooks.

This is great to prep ahead of time so, when you walk in the door at the end of the day, all you have to do is pop it in the oven.

Cover with aluminum foil and bake for 1 hour, then turn heat down to 375° F and cook uncovered for an additional 30 minutes, or until potatoes are tender.

Let stand for a few minutes before serving. Leftovers are wonderful!

RECIPES FOR AUTUMN

Fried Green Tomatoes Topped with Cheese on Pasta

What to do with all the green tomatoes on the vine as the growing season ends? Fried Green Tomatoes! *Green tomatoes are slightly sour and less sweet and juicy than ripened tomatoes but are delicious breaded and fried!*

- **1 bag gluten-free breadcrumbs**
- **2 farm-fresh eggs**
- **8 medium-sized green tomatoes**
- **frying oil**
- **basil**
- **oregano**
- **gluten-free pasta**
- **fresh grated Parmesan or Romano cheese**
- **2 cloves garlic**
- **½ cup olive oil**
- **½ tsp salt**

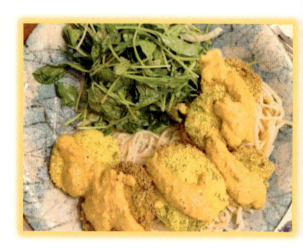

DIRECTIONS

Slice tomatoes into ½ inch thick slices.

Beat eggs in a bowl and set aside.

Pour breadcrumbs into another bowl and mix in fresh minced herbs and salt.

Heat oil in large frying pan until sizzling.

Dip tomato slices in egg, then coat in breadcrumbs, and place carefully in the hot oil.

RECIPES FOR AUTUMN

Reduce heat to medium-low and allow tomatoes to brown lightly on each side.

Drain tomatoes on a paper towel, then place on a cookie sheet in a warm oven (150–200° F).

Cook pasta, drain in colander, and return to pot.

Toss pasta in minced garlic and olive oil until well coated, then serve on plates. Place 3–4 slices of fried green tomatoes on pasta and top with grated cheese.

Goes great with a side of steamed greens or a fresh spinach salad.

RECIPES FOR AUTUMN

Roasted Pumpkin on Rice

Pumpkins are food, not just decoration, and this simple nutritious meal will have you looking at these seasonal gourds in a whole new way.

medium sized pumpkin (3–6 lbs), deseeded
   (save the seeds for roasting)
pumpkin seeds, roasted
brown rice
4 Tbsp butter, melted
1 Tbsp honey
½ tsp balsamic vinegar
½ cup hot water

DIRECTIONS

Roasting the Pumpkin Seeds: Remove pumpkin seeds and then peel the whitish hulls off their inner kernels (this is a great activity for the kids). Discard the hulls.

Toss pumpkin seeds in half of the melted butter, then lay on a cookie sheet and roast in a 300° F oven for 30 minutes (stir occasionally).

Set seeds aside.

Roasting the Pumpkin: Increase oven heat to 400° F and place hollowed out pumpkin on a cookie sheet and cook for about 30–45 min.

Slice pumpkin into wedges and then into chunks.

Return to the oven for another 15 minutes to brown further.

While the pumpkin is roasting, cook brown rice.

Honey Sauce: Whisk together remaining melted butter, hot water, balsamic vinegar, and honey.

Serve: Place roasted pumpkin on plates of rice, drizzle honey sauce on top, then sprinkle with the roasted pumpkin seeds. A side of steamed greens finishes the meal.

RECIPES FOR AUTUMN

Oven Roasted Brussels Sprouts

If you think you don't like Brussels sprouts, this easy recipe will change your mind. Makes a great entrée or side dish autumn through winter!

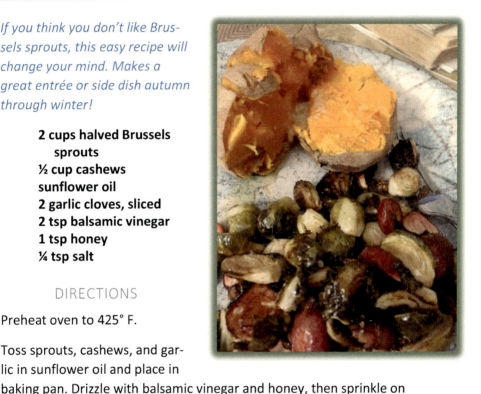

- 2 cups halved Brussels sprouts
- ½ cup cashews
- sunflower oil
- 2 garlic cloves, sliced
- 2 tsp balsamic vinegar
- 1 tsp honey
- ¼ tsp salt

DIRECTIONS

Preheat oven to 425° F.

Toss sprouts, cashews, and garlic in sunflower oil and place in baking pan. Drizzle with balsamic vinegar and honey, then sprinkle on the salt.

Bake for 18 minutes. Keep an eye on it during the final minutes. There should be a little charring along the edges—it enhances flavor and texture—but avoid scorching or the flavor will be ruined.

Tip: To prepare with sweet potato (pictured), prick sweet potato(es) several times with a fork or knife, then place on middle rack of 425° F oven, leaving room for the pan of sprouts. Large sweet potatoes take about 35 to 40 minutes to bake, so place pan of Brussels sprouts in oven about 15-20 minutes after starting the sweet potatoes.

Recipes for Autumn

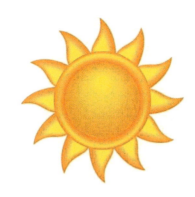

Meals for Any Season

MEALS FOR ANY SEASON

♥ Rice & Black Beans with Salsa

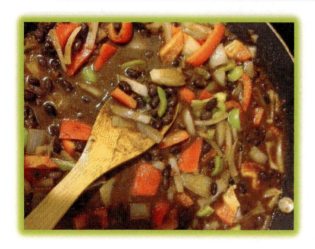

2 cans of black beans
4 cups cooked brown rice
1 medium onion
2 Tbsp Old Bay Seasoning
1 Tbsp garlic powder
1 jar of homemade salsa
   (see options below)

Summer Salsa

Chop *fresh* tomatoes, onion and peppers to make your own salsa and add cilantro.

Winter/Spring Salsa

Use roasted peppers and canned tomatoes put up from last season.

Tip: For salsa that resembles store-bought flavor, add a splash of red wine vinegar and salt to taste.

DIRECTIONS

In a large fry pan, add beans with onion powder, Old Bay, and salsa (or roasted peppers), then simmer on medium-low heat for about 20 minutes.

Serve bean concoction on top of rice with a seasonal side, if desired.

Side Option 1: Serve with hot buttered corn-on-the-cob and a garden-fresh salad.

Side Option 2: Serve with steamed greens (like chard, kale, or spinach).

MEALS FOR ANY SEASON

Indian Kitchari with Cucumber Salad

3 cups of red lentils
½ cup or more Panch Puran spice blend (cumin, fenugreek seeds, yellow mustard seeds, fennel seeds)
1 medium onion, minced
2 cloves garlic, minced
3 carrots, chopped

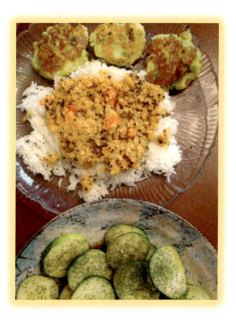

DIRECTIONS

Simmer lentils in water until soft, about 15–20 minutes. Set aside.

In a saucepan add about 2 Tbsp cooking oil and a packet of Panch Puran spices. Cook on medium heat until they are crackling and popping.

Add garlic, onion and carrots to the spices and continue to simmer.

Add the lentils and mix well to allow the lentils to absorb all the flavor.

Cover, simmer on low until carrots are tender (about 10–15 minutes).

Serve on brown rice with side of Aloo Tiki (see next page) and/or a simple cucumber salad (below).

Spice alternative: If you can't use Panch Puran spice blend, instead add a 2 tsp each curry powder and cumin and 1 Tbsp turmeric.

Cucumber Salad

2–3 large cucumbers, sliced
1 Tbsp honey
½ cup red wine vinegar
fresh dill

DIRECTIONS

Mix vinegar and honey until well blended. Pour over cucumber and allow to marinate. Garnish with fresh dill and a dash of salt.

MEALS FOR ANY SEASON

♥ Aloo Tikki (Indian Potato Cakes)

Makes about 12 cakes.

    4 medium-large potatoes
    ¾ cup organic peas
    1 medium carrot, diced fine
    3 Tbsp finely chopped cilantro
    1 Tbsp finely chopped coriander
    1 tsp curry powder

DIRECTIONS

Boil potatoes until cooked.

Add all the ingredients into a large bowl along with potatoes and mash well.

Form into palm sized patties (about 2½ to 3 inches across).

Oil a griddle or fry pan and fry up the aloo tikkis until brown and crisp.

Serve as a snack or as a side with lentils.

Top with green chutney.

Green Chutney

    2 cups chopped mint leaves
    1 cup chopped coriander
    1 large onion minced
    1 Tbsp lemon juice
    4 green chilies, chopped
    ½ inch piece of fresh ginger root, minced

Put all ingredients into a blender and puree. Spoon over aloo tikkis as a condiment.

Meals for Any Season

Tomato-Garlic Pasta

This is one of my all-time favorite quick meals!

1 pkg gluten-free pasta

4 fresh tomatoes, sliced into chunks *OR* a jar of put-up tomato sauce

2 cloves garlic, minced

½ cup olive oil

fresh basil, if available

DIRECTIONS

Cook pasta as directed.

Drain and rinse in cool water.

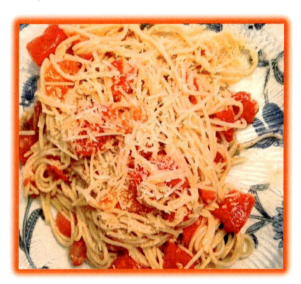

Return pasta to pot on low heat and toss in olive oil and garlic, blending well.

Finally, add tomatoes and lightly toss onto plates.

Salt to taste and garnish with fresh basil.

Option 1: Sprinkle with Parmesan cheese (as pictured).

Option 2: Mix in a cup of pesto (see recipe on page 88).

MEALS FOR ANY SEASON

♥ Chicky Cakes with Roasted Potatoes

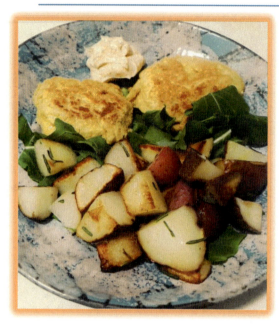

2 cans chickpeas,
   drained and rinsed
½ cup potato flour
2 Tbsp Vegannaise
   or mayonnaise
½ cup nutritional yeast
1 tsp hot mustard
2 stalks of celery diced
½ an onion diced
salt to taste
cooking oil

DIRECTIONS

Preheat oven to 425° F and prep potatoes first. Get them in the oven and then move on to the Chicky Cakes.

Mix together chickpeas, mayo, mustard, flour and nutritional yeast with a hand blender or food processor until the chickpeas are pretty broken up but not smooth. You may need to add more flour or mayo depending on texture—it should stick together, but not be too gooey.

Stir in diced celery and onion, then form batter into cakes.

Heat a pan of cooking oil until popping, then place patties into hot pan.

Lower heat to medium/medium-low and fry evenly on both sides.

Roasted Potatoes

2 sweet potatoes or 4 red potatoes cut in wedges

Toss in olive oil and salt with fresh minced rosemary

Roast in a 425° F oven until soft and browned, about 30 minutes.

MEALS FOR ANY SEASON

Portabella Mushroom Melt

1 large local portabella
   mushroom per person
2 cloves garlic, minced
½ cup or more Bragg's Liquid
   Aminos or soy sauce
Swiss cheese
local whole grain bread
   or GF bread, or brown rice
1 large bag of local greens
   (spinach, kale, or chard)

DIRECTIONS

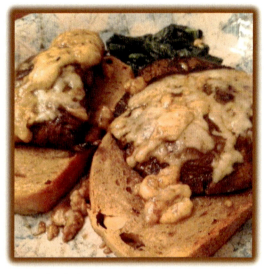

Preheat Oven to 400° F.

Marinate portabella caps in garlic and Bragg's or soy sauce for at least 30 minutes in a large casserole dish.

Cover dish with aluminum foil and roast in oven for about 20 minutes.

Uncover and add a slice of cheese over each mushroom.

Continue to cook uncovered another 10 minutes to melt the cheese.

Serve portabellas on bread or rice. You can also make sandwiches with caramelized onions added.

Steam greens as a side.

One of my daughter's all-time favorites!

Variation: During summer, top the mushrooms with sautéed onions and peppers with a side salad.

MEALS FOR ANY SEASON

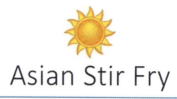

Asian Stir Fry

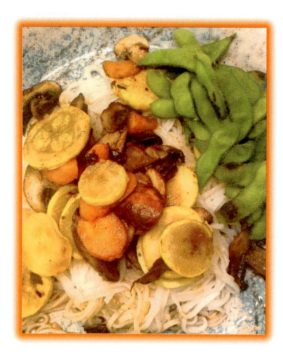

1 zucchini
2 yellow squash
1 medium onion
2 cloves of garlic, minced
2 carrots
1 cup sliced local mushrooms
1 bok choy
1–2 ichiban eggplants
1 pkg Asian rice noodles
2-inch chunk of ginger root, minced
½ cup or more Bragg's Liquid Aminos *or* soy sauce

Note: Substitute whatever veggies are available for your season—*get creative!* Also consider adding cubed local GMO-free tofu, tempeh, or a can of black beans

DIRECTIONS

Slice veggies into medallions or julienne-style and stir-fry on medium-high heat in a wok or large fry pan with a tsp each of vegetable and sesame oil.

Cook noodles according to package directions (or opt for rice instead).

When veggies start to soften, add the Bragg's Liquid Aminos (or soy sauce), ginger and garlic, and about 1 cup of water. Stir well.

Serve noodles or rice with stir fried veggies on top with a little of the sauce spooned over.

Suggestion: Try a side of steamed GMO-free edamame with a little saucer for dipping in Bragg's or soy sauce.

MEALS FOR ANY SEASON

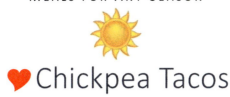

♥ Chickpea Tacos

1–2 avocados, pitted and diced
1 can chickpeas, drained
1 cup or more salsa
1–2 cups of fresh cilantro and salad greens, sliced fine
GMO-free taco shells (kids eat about 2 each and adults eat up to 4 each)
shredded cheddar cheese (optional)
1 tsp chili powder
½ tsp cumin
1 tsp garlic powder or 1 clove garlic, minced

DIRECTIONS

Preheat Oven to 250° F.

Place taco shells on cookie sheet and let warm in oven to crispen.

Place diced avocado and chickpeas in a bowl and mash well.

Add spices and mix to blend.

Carefully fill the hot shells with lettuce-cilantro mix, a spoonful of chickpea mixture, finally top with salsa and cheese.

MEALS FOR ANY SEASON

♥ Cheesy Quesadillas with Corn and Refried Black Beans

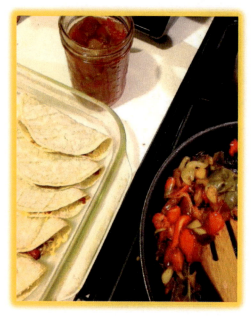

This is a huge hit with kids and can be modified many ways.

2 cans refried black beans
1 pkg corn or flour tortillas
1 Tbsp garlic powder
1 tsp chili powder
1 jar homemade salsa
2 cups shredded cheddar
corn on/off the cob (if off-cob, about ½ cup per person)

DIRECTIONS

Preheat oven to 350° F.

Warm tortillas in microwave for about 30 seconds per stack of six (this makes them less brittle and easier to fold without breaking).

Sprinkle about ¼ cup cheese on each wrap and fold in half. Place on cookie sheet. Place full sheets in oven for about 10–15 minutes.

In a medium pan warm beans mixed with salsa, garlic and chili powders. Stir occasionally. Remove from heat when bubbling.

Serve cheesy quesadillas on the plate with a hefty spoonful of refried beans and corn as sides.

Have homemade salsa available in dishes for dipping.

Variation: Sauté peppers and onion to add into the quesadilla along with the beans and cheese (pictured).

MEALS FOR ANY SEASON

♥ Nachos

Makes for a great lunch or quick dinner.

GMO-free local corn chips, large bag (if preferred, opt for a corn-free variety, like bean chips)
1–2 cans refried black beans
½ can of water
1–2 tsp cumin
1 large jar of salsa
2 cups shredded cheddar cheese
diced yellow, purple or green peppers (if in season)

DIRECTIONS

Preheat Oven to 350° F.

In a medium saucepan heat up the refried beans with cumin and water until a nice thick smooth consistency—not too watery but spreadable.

On 2 cookie sheets put a thick even layer of chips.

Spread the refried beans evenly across the chips.

Top with salsa and cheese.

Bake for about 20 minutes until the cheese melts.

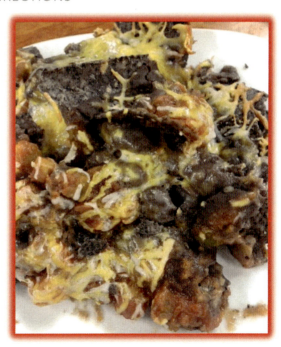

Barbecue Tofu or Tempeh with Roasted Veggies on Rice

- **1 block local GMO-free tofu or tempeh**
- **1 medium onion, sliced**
- **2 bell peppers, green and red, sliced** (fresh if in season or from your freezer from the previous summer)
- **3 cups cooked brown rice**

Barbecue Sauce

- **½ cup organic ketchup**
- **¼ cup Bragg's Liquid Aminos or soy sauce**
- **2 heaping Tbsp black strap molasses**
- **¼ cup balsamic vinegar**
- **1 Tbsp chili powder**
- **2 tsp garlic powder**
- **1 Tbsp Old Bay Seasoning**
- **1 cup water**
- **hot sauce to taste**

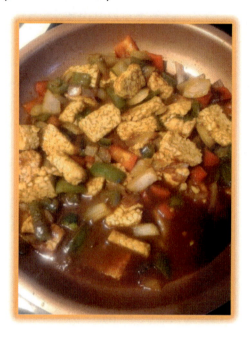

DIRECTIONS

Slice tofu or tempeh into steaks about ¼ inch thick and fry in 1 Tbsp veggie oil on medium high heat until golden brown on each side.

Cook Rice. 1½ cups rice to 3 cups water.

In a separate fry pan, cook up peppers and onions until soft.

Mix barbecue sauce ingredients.

Lay tofu on a bed of rice, top with veggies, and then generously spoon barbecue sauce on top.

Option: This also makes a great sandwich. Lay 2 slabs of fried tofu or tempeh on bread and drizzle with about 1 Tbsp sauce. Add sautéed onions and peppers. *Delicious!*

MEALS FOR ANY SEASON

Stuffed Baked Potatoes

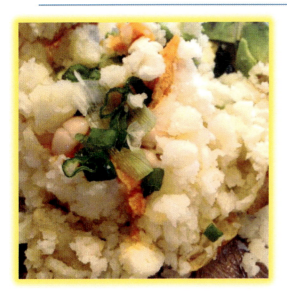

An easy, delicious meal to make!

1 large organic potato per person
1 medium onion, diced
1 can black beans
1 Tbsp Old Bay Seasoning
2-inch wedge of cheddar cheese, cubed or vegan cheese (p. 47)
1 stick of butter
1 head of broccoli (or other seasonal vegetables)

DIRECTIONS

Preheat oven to 400° F.

Wash potatoes and prick each several times with a knife then set directly on the oven rack. Bake for about 1 hour.

Warm black beans in a saucepan with a little Old Bay Seasoning.

Steam or sauté veggies in an uncovered saucepan until cooked. (Set aside some of the uncooked chopped onion for topping, if desired.)

Slice down the center of the cooked potato and open the center, using a fork rake over the potato to break it up.

Add the butter, veggies and black beans, then top with raw onion and cheese.

MEALS FOR ANY SEASON

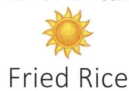

Fried Rice

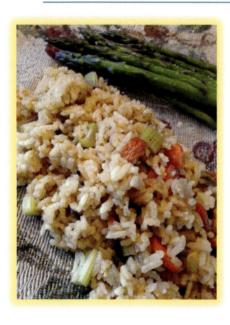

4 cups cooked rice
2 large stalks celery
2 large or 4 medium carrots
1 medium onion
1 Tbsp sesame oil
½ cup or more Bragg's Liquid Aminos *or* soy sauce
2-inch chunk ginger root, minced
2 cloves of garlic, minced
2 farm-fresh eggs (optional)

Option: *You can dice up squash, zucchini or broccoli, depending on what is in season. There are no rules as to what or how many vegetables you may use.*

DIRECTIONS

Cook rice by adding 2 cups rice into 4 cups boiling water, turn heat to low and cover. Done in 30–40 minutes.

Dice veggies and stir fry in sesame oil in wok or large frying pan on medium high heat until tender.

Fold in the rice and blend with a large cooking fork. Add the Bragg's Liquid Aminos (or soy sauce) and continue folding until well mixed.

Reduce heat to medium-low.

Egg option: *Make an indentation in the center of the wok, add the eggs, beat well, then fold into fried rice. Continue to fold and stir as the egg cooks.*

Serve with side of steamed asparagus in the spring, steamed greens in winter or fall, or a salad in summer. When steaming asparagus or greens, toss in sesame oil and add fresh sesame seeds to match the Asian theme.

MEALS FOR ANY SEASON

♥Cold Veggie Pasta Salad

pkg of GF pasta, cooked and cooled
local, seasonal veggies
   (for example: 1 head of broccoli, 2 medium heirloom tomatoes, 1 red pepper, 1 medium onion)
3 heaping Tbsp mayonnaise or Vegannaise
¼ cup red wine vinegar
fresh herbs: dill, basil, and/or oregano
salt to taste

DIRECTIONS

Dice raw veggies and toss into a bowl with the chilled pasta.

Add mayo, vinegar, salt, and minced herbs. Mix well.

A light, refreshing meal!

Option: Substitute a little finely chopped, steamed greens (as pictured) instead of broccoli.

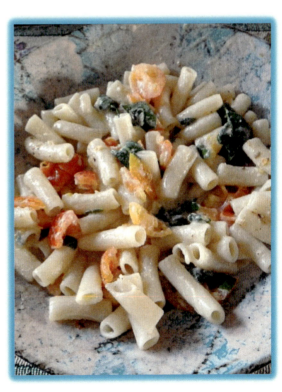

MEALS FOR ANY SEASON

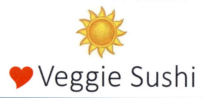

♥Veggie Sushi

This can be a fun family activity but sometimes a bit messy to prepare.

3 carrots
2 cucumber
1 cup shiitake mushrooms
1 large clove garlic, minced
2 ripe avocados
sticky rice (available at Asian markets)
rice vinegar
nori (seaweed rolling sheets)
pickled ginger
wasabi (Asian horseradish)
Bragg's or soy sauce

DIRECTIONS

Ingredient Preparation: Cook sticky rice HOURS before you are ready to roll. Put rice in a glass bowl and set in the fridge. Wait 2 Hours, lift and turn rice to release any heat. Continue to chill another hour.

Thinly slice the veggies, including the avocado.

Cook the mushrooms in garlic and Bragg's Liquid Aminos or Soy Sauce.

Place each of the prepared raw veggies on its own small plate.

Rolling: Have an open workspace for ingredients, nori, a small bowl of rice vinegar, and a platter for placing the finished wraps.

Start with a flat sheet of nori.

Dip fingertips in rice vinegar and take about 2–3 Tbsp sticky rice and spread along the center of the nori sheet.

Add some veggies along the rice (you can make single- and/or multi-veggie rolls, as you prefer).

MEALS FOR ANY SEASON

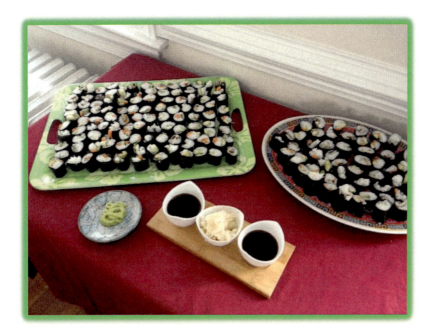

Roll the sheet until in a tight roll—*like a yoga mat!* If you're new to this craft, you can find sushi-rolling video tutorials online to give you a visualization how it's done.

Dip finger in rice vinegar and run wet finger along the edge of the sheet to "glue" the sushi roll in place.

Repeat until all the veggies and rice have been used.

Using a *very* sharp knife, carefully slice the sushi rolls into bite-sized pieces.

Serve: 6–8 pieces per person with small saucers of Bragg's Liquid Aminos or soy sauce for dipping, and pickled ginger slices, and a dab of wasabi (if preferred) on the side.

MEALS FOR ANY SEASON

♥Grandma Mary's Veggie Burgers

COURTESY OF MARY FIRESTONE FOORE

- **4 cups rolled oats**
- **2 cups cottage cheese**
- **3 Tbsp Bragg's Liquid Aminos** *or* **soy sauce**
- **1 cup pecan meal** (finely crushed pecans)
- **3 Tbsp powdered sage**
- **1 farm-fresh egg**
- **2 Tbsp nutritional yeast**
- **1 large chopped onion**
- **16 oz mushroom soup, creamy** (optional, as gravy)

DIRECTIONS

In a large bowl mix all the ingredients well.

Let mixture sit for about an hour (otherwise patties will fall apart).

Preheat oven to 350° F.

In a large fry pan add oil and heat on med-high until sizzling, then reduce heat to medium.

Form patties and carefully place into hot pan. Brown on each side (about 4–5 minutes). Transfer fried patties to a buttered casserole dish.

No gravy version: Bake in oven about 15 minutes, covered. After removing from oven, uncover and let cool five minutes before serving.

Gravy version: Pour cream of mushroom soup over patties. Bake *uncovered* in oven about 25 minutes.

Suggestions: These can be served as entrees (plain or with gravy), with toppings, or in sandwiches/burgers. The patties can also be diced and used in place of the vegan sausages in Shepherd's Pie (page 46).

Vegan Option: Omit the cottage cheese and eggs and replace them with ¼ cup oil, 3 Tbsp potato flour, ¼ cup cashews microwaved on high for 2 minutes in ¾ cup water, and ½ pound of silken tofu. Combine these ingredients together in a blender until smooth, then let sit 10 minutes.

MEALS FOR ANY SEASON

♥ Miso Soup with Fried Rice

Forget chicken noodle soup. This soup *is great for sinus issues and colds as it helps reduce mucous in the body. (And the chickens thank you.)*

- **½ container of GMO-free miso paste**
- **1 medium onion**
- **1–2 cups shiitake mushrooms**
- **1 block Twin Oaks GMO-free tofu, cubed**
- **½ stick of organic butter**

DIRECTIONS

Melt butter in a saucepan.

Slice onion and mushrooms and add to saucepan. Sauté until onion is translucent.

In a large pot add about 4–6 cups of water and bring to a boil.

Mash in the miso into the water pot until it is dissolved into a broth. Reduce heat to medium-low.

Add mushrooms, onions, and cubed tofu, then simmer to desired consistency, stirring occasionally.

Serve with Fried Rice (see page 68) on the side.

Note: This soup is also a great side or starter with other Asian dishes, like Veggie Sushi (page 70) or Asian Rice Noodle Stir Fry (page 48).

MEALS FOR ANY SEASON

Vegetarian Chili with Corn Bread

6–8 large tomatoes
   (seasonal in Virginia into October)
4 carrots
1½ cups corn (optional)
1 large onion
2 cloves garlic
2 cans kidney beans
2 cans black beans
1 cup diced local mushrooms
1 cup cooked brown rice

Seasoning Ingredients

2–3 Tbsp chili powder
2 Tbsp Old Bay Seasoning
¼ cup black strap molasses
¼ cup balsamic vinegar
¼ cup Bragg's Liquid Aminos
   or **soy sauce**
2 Tbsp Grey Poupon mustard

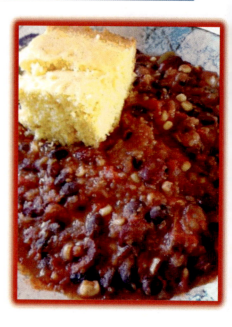

DIRECTIONS

Cut carrots, tomatoes, and onion into small chunks.

In a large pot add the tomatoes and simmer for 15 minutes, stirring occasionally until tomatoes begin to fall apart, making a chunky sauce.

Stir in remaining ingredients.

Now add the seasoning ingredients and stir to blend.

Simmer on low heat for about an hour.

Corn Bread: Prepare GF corn bread from mix according to box directions. Trader Joe's and Glutino are our favorite brands.

Variation: Enhance the corn bread by adding a pureed small yellow squash to the batter (adds moisture and it tastes great).

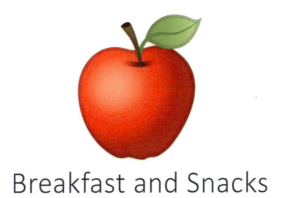

Breakfast and Snacks

BREAKFAST AND SNACKS

Breakfast at Ms. Nitya's

At my house, I eat oats every breakfast. In spring and summer, I enjoy homemade granola, often with fruit. In fall and winter, I have hot oatmeal or steel cut oats.

Spring & Summer Homemade Granola

- **6 scoops of bulk bin organic regular oats** (roughly 8 cups)
- **½ stick organic lightly salted butter**
- **1 cup of local honey**
- **½ cup molasses** (optional)
- **1 cup walnut pieces**
- **½ cup raw sunflower seeds**
- **1 cup dried fruit**

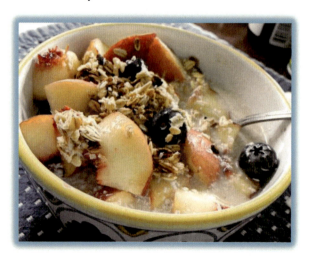

DIRECTIONS

Preheat oven to 450° F.

Melt butter with honey and molasses on low heat, stirring gently.

Place oats with seeds and nuts in a large bowl.

Mix in the melted butter, honey and molasses with a wooden spoon until the oats are thoroughly coated.

Spread the oat mix *evenly* onto a large baking sheet and bake for no more than 8 minutes (you do NOT want to scorch the oats).

Breakfast and Snacks

Turn the oven off and crack the oven door open. Allow the oats to continue to dry in the warm oven as they slowly cool. Use a spatula to lift the oats off the tray and into a storage container.

Toss in 1 cup of dried fruit (chopped dates, raisins, cranberries, etc.).

Cooking Variations: Replace the last 3 ingredients with 2 Tbsp Pumpkin Pie Spice and 1 cup raw pumpkin seeds or 1 Tbsp cinnamon and 1 cup of pecan pieces.

Serving Variations: Top your bowl with any dried or seasonal fresh fruit or berries, banana, and/or coconut.

Be creative! Come up with your own variations!

Autumn & Winter Hot Oats with Fruit

Serves 2 people.

- **1 cup nut milk** (enough to cover the oats)
- **1 cup regular *or* steel cut oats**
- **¼ cup nut pieces** (walnuts and pecans are my favorites)
- **¼ cup raisins or other dried fruit** (like home-canned peaches, diced apple pieces, or a sliced banana)

DIRECTIONS

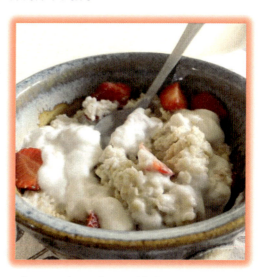

Heat the milk until just boiling, reduce heat to low, then add the oats.

Cook time for steel-cut oats 45–60 min; regular oats 10–15 minutes. If oats start to dry out before finished, add a little water.

Serve with a dollop of local yogurt and a drizzle of local honey or blackstrap molasses.

BREAKFAST AND SNACKS

Fruit Smoothie (dessert)

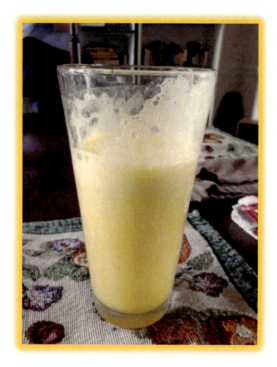

2 large bananas (peeled)
6 peaches (peeled, pitted)
6 oranges (peeled, deseeded)
2 cups local organic plain yogurt (optional)

DIRECTIONS

In a blender whiz up the ingredients while adding 1 to 2 handfuls of ice cubes to chill.

Pour and enjoy!

BREAKFAST AND SNACKS

Green Juice Cleanse

Spring is a great time to try replacing one meal for a raw juice. Investing in a good juicer is so worth the benefits to your health. Get inspired by watching the documentary Fat, Sick, and Nearly Dead.

8 kale leaves
1 bunch of swiss chard
4–6 carrots (with some greens, if in good condition, well rinsed)
4 celery stalks
2 beets (with some greens, if in good condition, well rinsed)
1 apple
2-inch, finger-thick piece of ginger root

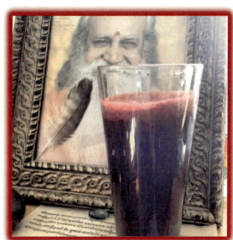

Liquefy in a juicer. If you don't have one, you can use a blender, then filter out excess fiber using a wire mesh strainer over a large bowl.

SUGGESTIONS

Get creative! Add whatever other raw foods you'd like. I prefer adding extra ginger.

If you struggle with the bitterness of the greens, don't reduce them! They provide the ultimate in vitamins, minerals, and antioxidants. Instead, add an extra apple—it really softens the bite!

If you store leftover juice, keep it from sunlight and make sure you drink it within 24 hours (48 if refrigerated). This is to prevent enzymes and other vital nutrients from degrading.

Tip: Stored juice will settle. Shake or stir before pouring.

BREAKFAST AND SNACKS

Fruit Juice Cleanse

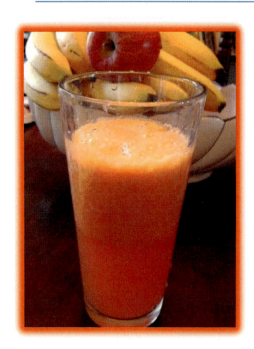

Keep in mind that a large fruit juice is going to give you a huge surge in natural sugar. This should not be a problem as long as you burn it off. Plan on an active morning (Hatha Yoga, a meditative walk, a hike, bike ride or a good swim) to put that energy to use. The exertion will also help pump those antioxidants through your body and eliminate toxins and wastes. Think of the juice as your cleaner, your exercise is the scrubbing, and drinking water throughout the day as your system's rinse.

2 apples
2–4 *sustainable* **bananas**
2–4 peeled oranges
4 carrots
1–2 cups fresh strawberries, washed with tops
   (in season from late April into early June)
1 cup thawed blueberries
   (picked last summer and frozen in freezer bags)

Liquefy in a juicer. If you don't have one, you can use a blender, then filter out excess fiber using a wire mesh strainer over a large bowl.

SUGGESTIONS

You can really play with what you have available and what's in season.

A pineapple can be another fun addition.

If you store leftover juice, refrigerate and be sure you drink it within 24 hours.

BREAKFAST AND SNACKS

♥Yogi Yum-Yums (snack)

Serves 8. *This is a different recipe from the one I originally made at camp. This one is far cheaper, easier, and with fewer ingredients.*

- **1½ cups chopped dates**
- **½ cup fresh ground peanut butter** (or sunbutter or almond butter)
- **½ cup rolled oats**
- **2–3 Tbsp chocolate protein powder** (Orgain brand is GMO-free, soy free, gluten-free, and sugar-free)

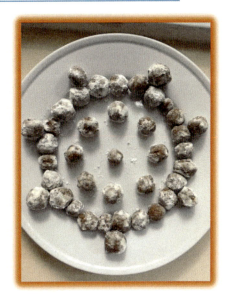

DIRECTIONS

Put all the ingredients into a food processor and blend *two minutes*, at which point mixture will become well blended.

Spoon into a bowl and roll into one-inch balls.

Tip: The mixture should seem dry, but if balls don't hold together, return to food processor and blend in 1 Tbsp coconut oil to make them more malleable.

Variation 1: Roll balls in shredded coconut for an added treat.

Variation 2: You can also roll balls in sunflower seeds.

Suggestion: Serve 2–3 balls with a fruit, such as a slice of cantaloupe, peach, or apple, depending on the season.

BREAKFAST AND SNACKS

Chickpea Poppers (snack)

A great popcorn alternative and way more nutritious!

    2 cans of chickpeas drained and left to dry in sieve
    2 tsp cumin
    2 tsp garlic powder
    1 tsp olive oil

DIRECTIONS

Preheat oven to 350° F.

Mix all ingredients well and spread onto a cookie sheet.

Bake for 45 min.

Ultimate Rice Cake (snack)

    Plain or cinnamon rice cake
    Raisins, berries *or* sliced peaches *or* thinly sliced apples
        (depending on the season)
    Nut *or* seed butter

Spread nut or seed butter on rice cake and add toppers. Our favorite at yoga camp is sliced peaches and a few blueberries.

Breakfast and Snacks

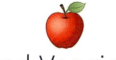

Fruit and Veggie Snacks

Apple Slices with Nut or Seed Butter

Local organic apple sliced to dip in fresh ground nut or seed butter OR a great travel snack is to core the apple and fill with nut or seed butter.

Hummus with Veggies

>   **1 can of chickpeas drained**
>   **2 tbsp tahini**
>   **¼ cup water**
>   **1 clove of pressed garlic**
>   **2 tbsp olive oil**
>   **salt to taste**
>   **squeeze of lemon *or* chili paste if desired**

Mix all ingredients until super smooth. Dip with your favorite sliced veggies (rigid vegetables, such as celery, carrot sticks, sliced peppers, or cucumber slices) and enjoy!

Variations: Serve with pita chips or warmed pita bread, use as a sandwich spread, or toss into pasta with olives and chopped spinach.

Yogurt with Fruit and Granola

Single serving:

>   **½ cup local plain yogurt**
>   **½ cup homemade granola** (see recipe page 76)
>   **½ cup diced fruit of the season: peaches, berries, or bananas**

In a soup size bowl add the yogurt, then top with granola, then fruit and/or berries.

Breakfast and Snacks

♥ Zucchini Muffins (dessert)

Makes 24 muffins. **Note:** You can make your own oat flour by simply whizzing oats for several seconds in a blender or coffee grinder.

- **2 medium zucchinis**
- **1½ cups gluten-free flour**
- **⅔ cup oat flour**
- **1 tsp baking soda**
- **1½ tsp baking powder**
- **½ tsp salt**
- **2 tsp cinnamon**
- **½ cup organic brown sugar**
- **1 cup organic raisins**
- **½ cup coconut oil**
- **4 farm-fresh eggs**
- **½ cup almond milk**

DIRECTIONS

Preheat oven to 350° F.

Grease muffin tins.

Shred zucchini in a food processor using the grater attachment (or grate by hand).

Lay zucchini out on a hand towel, then roll the towel and twist firmly to squeeze out any moisture.

In a large bowl put the flour, oat flour, baking soda, baking powder, salt, and cinnamon and blend well with a wooden spoon.

Add the brown sugar and mix to remove any lumps.

Make a well in the middle of the flour bowl and add the coconut oil (slightly warmed until melted), eggs, and almond milk.

Beat egg mixture well into dry ingredients, then fold in the shredded zucchini, followed by the raisins

Option: If desired, at this point add chopped nuts and/or blueberries.

Mix batter thoroughly, then spoon into muffin tins about ⅔ full.

Bake 20 minutes. Cool before removing from the tins. Refrigerate leftovers to prevent spoilage.

Breakfast and Snacks

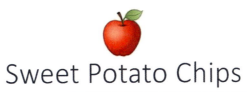

Sweet Potato Chips

2 sweet potatoes, *very* **thinly sliced**
1 tsp cinnamon *or* **curry powder**
¼ cup vegetable oil
½ tsp salt

Preheat Oven to 400° F.

Put ingredients in a bowl and toss until covered.

Place evenly on a cookie sheet, and roast about 20 minutes until crispy.

BREAKFAST AND SNACKS

♥ Strawberry Crumble (dessert)

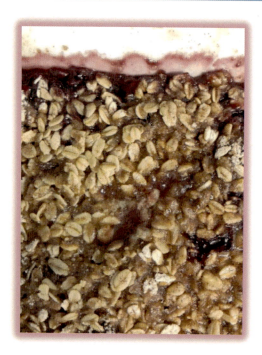

4–6 cups local strawberries
1 cup organic sugar
1 cup organic brown sugar
1 cup gluten-free oats
½ cup gluten-free flour
5 Tbsp butter, softened

DIRECTIONS

Preheat oven to 325° F.

Slice strawberries, removing tops.

In a medium bowl, mix strawberries with white sugar and pour into a buttered 1½ quart casserole dish.

In a separate bowl combine brown sugar, oats, and flour, then cut in butter. Spoon this mixture over the strawberry mixture.

Bake for 45 minutes to 1 hour.

Variation: This recipe can also be made with apples, berries, or peaches (or combinations) when in season

Tip: For an extra treat, top with coconut milk ice cream.

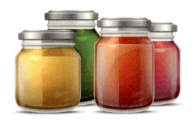

Putting Up for Winter

PUTTING UP FOR WINTER

Freezing Ingredients

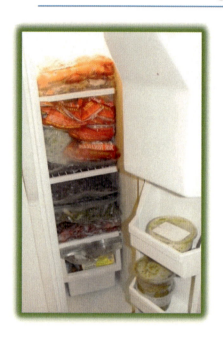

There are four general methods for preserving foods: dehydrating, canning, pickling, and freezing. Freezing is the simplest, and most freezers can hold a lot of preserved food to last you through the winter. This allows you to continue eating locally-sourced foods preserved from their peak season. So in January, you can enjoy the delight of blueberries in your hot oatmeal, or roasted peppers in your quesadillas.

These are some of my favorite foods to have in my freezer for the winter months.

Pesto

MODIFIED FROM *MOOSEWOOD RESTAURANT COOKS AT HOME* COOKBOOK BY THE MOOSEWOOD COLLECTIVE.

I make this in the summer when basil is in abundance, and so for the purpose of freezing multiple batches for winter, this recipe is *six times* a standard recipe. Reuse small plastic containers (like from store-bought hummus or feta cheese) to freeze dinner-size portions to enjoy off-season.

- **12 cups loosely packed basil leaves**
- **18 cloves of local garlic minced**
- **3 cups of extra virgin olive oil**
- **3 cups grated Parmesan** (optional—perfectly yummy without it)
- **4 cups pine nuts** (or chopped walnuts for a cheaper alternative)

DIRECTIONS

Divide the ingredients into thirds so you can run several batches through your food processor.

Process until smooth.

There is *nothing* like freshly made pesto tossed into GF pasta and topped with cubed heirloom tomatoes. *So rich, so creamy, so yummy!*

Roasted Veggies

The peak of summer is when you want to hit the farmer's market and buy in bulk. Many farmers offer deals in late July and early August when they have more than they can sell.

I buy in large quantities the following to roast.

12 eggplants
12 red peppers
24 green peppers
12 yellow peppers
12–24 zucchinis
48 or more tomatoes (plum, heirloom, and/or red)
12 large onions
olive oil
sea salt
3 cups fresh basil

DIRECTIONS

Preheat oven to 450° F. Slice these veggies.

Place veggies on a cookie sheet and toss in olive oil and a little sea salt.

Roast for about 30 minutes. Watch out that they don't burn! Continue until all veggies have been roasted.

Now make your "future meals" as you fill up your half gallon freezer bags (see bag-sealing directions on p. 80). Some bags should be tomatoes (with sprigs of basil for zest), others will be mixed roasted veggies (your preferred combinations of eggplant, zucchini, tomatoes, onions, and peppers with a few sprigs of basil or other herbs).

PUTTING UP FOR WINTER

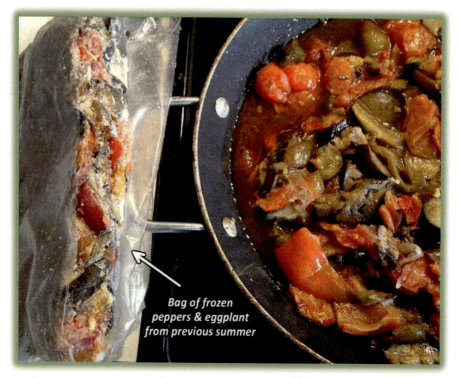

Bag of frozen peppers & eggplant from previous summer

When you take these stored treasures out of the freezer months later and defrost for cooking, use them whole as toppings on pasta or rice, or in stews, or puree the tomatoes for smooth soups or sauces.

From any of the roasted veggie bags you can easily break off the amount you want (don't think you have to use the whole bag), then just reseal and put the remainder back in the freezer.

PUTTING UP FOR WINTER

How to Seal Your Freezer Bags

Fill bag 80% full and lay it flat on the counter.

Zip the bag until nearly closed.

Put your mouth over the small opening and suck deeply to pull ANY remaining air out—the bag should look shrunken—quickly seal the bag completely closed.

Lay bags flat in the freezer. You'll be surprised how well these stack (I sometimes get them ten high). Make sure the outsides are dry or the bags will stick together when frozen.

Blueberries

Make a trip to Swift Creek Berry Farm or another pick-it-yourself blueberry farm in July and pick 3 to 4 full buckets.

Dump berries into a strainer. Rinse and clean out stems and leaves.

Allow them to dry spread out on cotton hand towels.

Roll the blueberries into quart-size Ziploc bags and follow sealing directions (above).

Peaches

If you want to avoid the time-consuming mess of canning, you can easily freeze peaches.

Scald the peaches in boiling water for one minute, then slip skins off.

Slice peaches and toss in organic sugar.

Scoop the peaches into quart-size Ziploc bags and follow sealing directions (above).

You can also make *Peach Pie Filling*:

4–6 cups sliced peaches
1 cup organic sugar
¼ cup GF flour
1 tsp cinnamon
2 Tbsp lemon juice (fresh from the lemon)

PUTTING UP FOR WINTER

Simply toss peaches in other ingredients (add blueberries, if you like). Freeze as described on previous page.

Now you can make fresh local peach pie for a holiday surprise or a treat on a snowy winter night.

Corn

Enjoy sweet corn all year long! At peak season buy several dozen ears of corn. Cut corn off the cob RAW. Place in quart-size resealable bags.

Following sealing direction from previous page.

Grated Zucchini

A great use for those oversized end of season zucchinis is to grate them in a food processor. Put in a large strainer in the sink for several hours to drain excess moisture.

Seal in bags for making muffins (page 84), Crabby Cakes (page 30) or adding to soups during the winter months.

What else?

The freezing process can damage the texture of some foods, but you learn best from experience—so experiment with small quantities of your favorite foods before trying bulk volumes. Strawberries often become spongey and tasteless after freezing. You'd do better to make jam or jelly. Okra is another one that doesn't do well by itself but can be roasted with other vegetables.

Zucchini bread (can substitute peaches or apples too) works well. Bake 12 mini loaves and wrap in aluminum foil, then store in reused tortilla wrap bags or freezer bags.

Putting Up for Winter

A Word About Canning

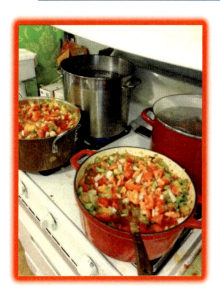

If you are new to canning, the good news is that there are numerous how-to videos and lessons online for free. Canning isn't rocket science, but you do not want to get it wrong. I have lost a batch of salsa because the jars didn't seal correctly.

Best is to get a bulk supply of ingredients when they're in season. Roma tomatoes are favorites because they make the best sauce.

If you have a dishwasher you can sterilize the jars that way, otherwise you'll need to boil them in a large pot of water.

This is an all-day event and very messy. Have available hand towels and make sure your work surfaces are clear of clutter. You will need a canning kit that includes a funnel, magnetic wand, and canning tongs. So, do like I do and turn up the music and make it super fun!

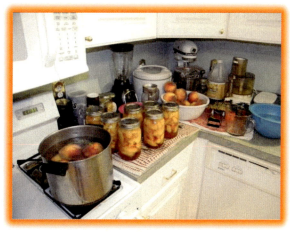

There is a rhythm to the process, and it can be a meditative experience. You can't beat the feeling of satisfaction when it's all done and there are dozens of jars full of top-quality sauces ready for winter. It's also less wasteful because only the lids are replaced each season—the jars can be reused for many years

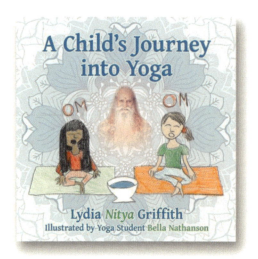
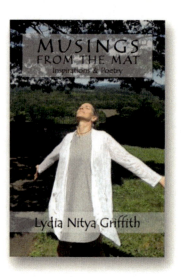

A Child's Journey into Yoga
Paperback, Color, 4th–6th Grade Reading Level
Based on the Yoga Sutras of Patanjali, this story follows the life of Mica as she learns to live an ethical life. Far beyond the physical poses, yoga teaches us how to be healthy in body, mind, and spirit. This story will inspire young yogis to stay the course on their inward journey toward self-knowledge and inner peace.

Musings from the Mat
Paperback, 6" x 9", 170 pages
Selected from newsletters, blogs and poetry going back to 2000, this exquisitely inspired compilation is deeply personal, raw, and authentic. Nitya's writing takes you on a spiritual yogi's journey through life with wisdom and profound understanding of the human narrative.

Nitya Living Yoga Camps
for kids & teens
Established in 2005 and regionally renowned, these full-day camp programs teach children how to live yoga through fun activities, crafts, outdoor adventures, meditation, self-inquiry, and practicing compassion.

Nitya Living Yoga Teacher Training
Certification to teach 2 to 16-year-olds mindfulness Yoga that supports SEL (social-emotional learning) practices. Training is available throughout the USA.

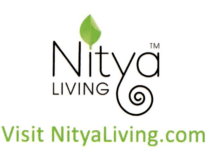

Visit NityaLiving.com

Made in the USA
Middletown, DE
05 June 2021